D0163893

The Essential Guide to Managing Consultants

Strategies for Healthcare Leaders

The Essential Guide to Managing Consultants

Strategies for Healthcare Leaders

by Michael E. Rindler

Health Administration Press
Chicago, IL

Your board, staff, or clients may also benefit from this book's insight. For more information on quantity discounts, contact the Health Administration Press Marketing Manager at (312) 424-9470.

This publication is intended to provide accurate and authoritative information in regard to the subject matter covered. It is sold, or otherwise provided, with the understanding that the publisher is not engaged in rendering professional services. If professional advice or other expert assistance is required, the services of a competent professional should be sought.

The statements and opinions contained in this book are strictly those of the author(s) and do not represent the official positions of the American College of the Healthcare Executives or of the Foundation of the American College of Healthcare Executives.

Copyright © 2002 by the Foundation of the American College of Healthcare Executives. Printed in the United States of America. All rights reserved. This book or parts thereof may not be reproduced in any form without written permission of the publisher.

06   05   04   03   02   5   4   3   2   1

Library of Congress Cataloging-in-Publication Data

Rindler, Michael.
   The essential guide to managing consultants: strategies for healthcare leaders/
   by Michael E. Rindler.
      p. cm.
   Includes bibliographical references.
   ISBN 1-56793-192-8
   1. Hospital consultants. 2. Health services administrators. 3. Leadership.
   4. Hospitals—Administration. I. Title.

   RA 971 .R5385 2002
   362.1'1—dc21

                                                              2002068563

The paper used in this publication meets the minimum requirements of American National Standard for Information Sciences—Permanence of Paper for Printed Library Materials, ANSI Z39.48-1984. ⊚ ™

Acquisitions editor: Audrey Kaufman; Project manager: Cami Cacciatore;
Book designer: Matt Avery; Cover designer: Betsy Pérez

Health Administration Press
A division of the Foundation of the
   American College of Healthcare Executives
1 North Franklin Street, Suite 1700
Chicago, IL 60606-3491
(312) 424-2800

Table of Contents

Foreword   vii

Preface   xi

Acknowledgments   xiii

PART ONE: FIVE KEYS TO CONSULTING SUCCESS

1   Knowing When to Use Consultants   3

2   Selecting the Best Consultant   17

3   Working Effectively with Consultants   33

4   Avoiding the Common Pitfalls   43

5   Taking Action: The Secret of Success   53

PART TWO: CONSULTANTS FOR GOVERNING BOARDS

6   Board Performance Improvement   65

7   Certified Public Accountants   79

8   Turnaround Consultants   93

9   Chief Executive Officer Search   103

10 Strategic Planning   117

11 Legal Consultation   129

PART THREE: CONSULTANTS TO MANAGEMENT

12 Improving Financial Performance   141

13 Improving Clinical Performance   153

14 Improving Customer Service   165

15 Marketing   175

16 Human Resources   187

17 Architects   197

18 Technology   207

19 Medical Staff Consultations   213

Afterword: The Ideal Consultant   225

APPENDICES

Appendix A: Sample Request for Proposal   229
Financial Performance Improvement

Appendix B: Sample Letter of Engagement   234
FinancialPerformance Improvement

Appendix C: Sample Request for Proposal   240
Governance Performance Improvement

Appendix D: Sample Governance Policy Manual Table of   246
Contents and Sample Policies

Appendix E: Sample Request for Proposal   260
Audit Services

Appendix F: Sample Request for Proposal   265
Legal Services

Appendix G: Sample Letter of Engagement   269
Human Resources Consultation

Appendix H: Sample Request for Proposal   274
Architectural Services

About the Author   281

Foreword

As I write this, many of our nation's hospitals are struggling financially. About a third of them are experiencing break-even operating margins, and there's red ink on the bottom line for another third. Margins have deteriorated since the Balanced Budget Act of 1997 put in place five years of Medicare funding cuts; while some relief was obtained from Congress in 1999 and 2000, many of those "fixes" are scheduled to expire unless further relief is provided.

At the same time, the skimping national economy has led employers to reduce health benefits and/or shift more fiscal responsibility to employees. The slump also has put significant pressures on state governments, leading to double-digit percentage cuts in some Medicaid program payments. Each of these realities has contributed to an increasing number of uninsured patients presenting at hospitals for care—usually at an emergency room that already is overextended as a shortage of nurses has strained the staffing of that department and the beds upstairs.

It's not a pretty financial picture for hospitals where unionization and employee-related expenses are on the rise, there is a disappearing market for professional liability insurance coverage, and physicians are "carving out" the more profitable services to shore up their own financial situation. As geographic markets and hospital margins become less stable, rating agencies and investors are more uncertain about hospital credit risks. Access to capital will be increasingly challenging at the same time that capacity is strained by an aging population with increasing incidence of chronic disease.

Given all of this, it's a time when, yet again, hospital leaders are inclined to look for assistance from the legions of consultants who serve the health sector.

From the early 1980s to the early 1990s, I was one of those consultants. It was the 10 years following Medicare's switch to a "prospective payment" system and uncertainty prevailed. Clients were calling for a variety of reasons, including the need to educate their governing boards, rethink their strategic plans, or bone up on the incentives and implications under capitation and other forms of fixed payments.

The initial call always was the most telling. In some cases, the client's stated need turned out to be right on target—well thought out and well integrated with a viable strategic plan. In a disturbing number of cases, while the client clearly understood the operative question, the proposed response—and therefore the proposed engagement—needed significant recrafting. And, in even more dramatic cases, the client only knew the question and had little clue what the necessary response might entail. "Client education" was needed even before a commitment to serve or referral to another consultant could be made.

I learned over those 10 years that consulting is greatly misunderstood and misused. As I was told once by a consultant at a seminar, "A consultant can tell you how to take a bath. He can even show you how. But, no matter what, he can never take the bath for you." In the worst of cases, people look to consultants to make up for a deficit in their ability or experience when they should be seeking to change fundamental behavior and operations with guidance from a consultant. If you can see that your current structure, skill deployment, and strategic initiatives are all contributing to the results being achieved, there is nothing else to do but institute fundamental changes in one or all of these domains. Anything less will be a "quick fix" at best, not a long-term solution.

It may seem backward, but the healthier your organization is, the more you are likely to get out of a consulting experience. That's because the culture of a healthy organization is already open to change; sometimes it's more difficult for a troubled organization to come to the conclusion that fundamental behavior changes are the only hope. It takes real leadership to admit that the current efforts are out of alignment and that only an outside perspective and complementary set of skills can help work out the particular problem.

In this book, Michael Rindler offers practical advice on selecting, engaging, and getting the most out of an experienced consultant. Contrary to the stereotype of a consultant, Michael doesn't sell first; rather, he cautions readers not to waste their money if they are not ready to use consultative services most effectively. An old joke applies here: "How many psychiatrists does it take to change a light bulb? Only one, but the light bulb really has to want to change!" Hospital leaders *really* have to want to change if the consulting engagement is targeted in a problem area.

I can see this even more clearly now as a multi-organizational system executive. Hospital executives are proud people, and rightly so. They have risen to meet the needs of their communities, and they run one of the most complicated community organizations imaginable. Hospitals are very quality oriented and it is not easy to admit that outside help may be needed. It can be disruptive, to say the least. Think about it: introducing a new person with new ideas into a culture and environment that does not know this person, that might have long-tenured team members and strong personalities of its own, and that may already have strong opinions about what needs to be done and how. A short-term and focused intervention, at dollar levels greater than anyone inside the organization will make in annual salary, will cause some strain. In addition, the better the consultant, the more she or he will expect the client to do between consultant visits to move the project along. This "homework" often entails the very work that the group has already tried to tackle once or more.

Yes, there are times when consultants are used for positive purposes rather than problem solving. Michael addresses such cases as well, as with architects to build a new facility or IT consultants to select and install an exciting new information system. While by nature happier and more future-oriented assignments, these consultations are not without stress either. Again, organizational culture plays a huge role—how much do people want a new facility or system to look and function like the one they now have? How open are they to new functions and capabilities? Some will see such a major undertaking as the crown jewel in their careers, a view that may not lead to collaborative planning and teamwork.

I have known Michael as both an accomplished hospital executive and as a consultant/author. This book portrays his personality and style quite nicely. He tells it like he has seen it. Michael has no tolerance for waste or subpar results. He doesn't like to be distracted from the basics until they are working most effectively. He believes in high standards, and client/consultant relationships are no exception because he has been on both sides. Read this book and take his advice: buy the best in integrity and experience, expect to pay for it, but understand the difference between the price of engagement (and potential solution) versus the cost of not addressing the opportunity for improvement. Understand that such payment is an investment in a better future; but, most of all, don't spend unless you are looking to make significant change.

—Richard J. Umbdenstock
President and CEO, Providence Services
Spokane, WA

Preface

A HIDDEN WINDFALL of dollars is available to the healthcare industry: more money for nurses' salaries, better fringe benefits for service workers, and improved facilities and technology. Where is this money hidden and how can you access it?

Healthcare organizations waste millions of dollars annually on consultants. Some waste both time and money by not recognizing opportunities or anticipating problems that could be successfully handled with the help of consultants. Others waste even more resources with poor consultant hiring practices or ineffective oversight. This book is designed to help healthcare leaders recognize when a consultant is needed, how and when to hire the best consultants, and how to achieve the best possible outcomes when consultants are retained. The windfall comes from eliminating the millions of dollars wasted on consultants.

Achieving the best results from a consulting engagement is a matter of practicing good management fundamentals. Part One of this book covers the five basics of working effectively with consultants. The next two parts go into detail concerning good practices for working with consultants to governing boards and consultants to management. The Afterword articulates the characteristics of an ideal consultant. Appendices provide practical examples of requests for proposals and engagement letters designed to get the optimum value from consulting dollars.

Key themes reinforced throughout the book encourage leaders to:

- Articulate the problem and desired outcome first.
- Consider internal resources as an alternative to consultants.

- Exercise due diligence in selecting the very best consultant available.
- Carefully oversee the consulting engagement.
- Listen to what the consultant says.
- Do something positive with the consultant's recommendations.

In my three decades of experience as a healthcare chief executive and healthcare consultant, I have seen tremendous amounts of money wasted on consultants by dysfunctional and ineffective healthcare leaders who hire unqualified consultants to accomplish poorly defined goals. The many examples throughout this book illustrating key points are all true stories, with some changes to protect the identities of the parties. Many of the examples are negative in character, providing insights about behaviors to avoid. Some of the examples are so bad you may conclude that they are stranger than fiction.

Achieving the best results with consultants requires capable, well-organized, and thoughtful management approaches. Much of this book is devoted to suggestions for improving management and governance. These topics are equally germane to hospitals, clinics, long-term care facilities, HMOs, and other healthcare organizations. Effective boards and management teams make excellent consulting clients if they are able to select the best consultants and make excellent use of their counsel. Poorly functioning boards or management teams are far less likely to use consulting advice effectively. This book offers many suggestions for improving governance and management, which provide a foundation for making the best use of consultants. If consultation becomes necessary, well-managed organizations achieve better results. However, even the most gifted consultants cannot help organizations led by inept boards and management teams.

The recently exposed breakdown of executive leadership and consulting practices at Enron, one of the largest corporate failures in history, illustrates why the strong language in this book is so appropriate. This book strives to offer candid and objective advice, not politically correct platitudes.

Avoid consultants if you can. If you can't, hire the best—not the most available, the cheapest, or the biggest. Hire the *best*. The fundamental message of this book is to hire the very best consultant when outside consultation is absolutely necessary. You will never be disappointed with the best.

—*Michael E. Rindler*

Acknowledgments

A CONSULTANT'S TRUE value is determined by the cumulative experiences he acquires in the course of his career. Consultants who have had the good fortune to work for insightful clients accumulate wisdom from them and the challenging assignments they offer. In my consulting career I have worked for over one hundred excellent clients. Seven offered defining experiences that inspired this book.

Lottie Kurcz, Chairman of the Board, Holy Cross Hospital, led her organization successfully through one of the most challenging governance, financial, and quality turnarounds ever attempted. Jim Kluttz, President, Frederick Memorial Healthcare, built one of the most successful independent community hospitals with quiet competence and great dignity. Steve Ronstrom, Administrator, Sacred Heart Hospital, used his remarkable intellect to create a hugely successful Catholic healthcare organization.

Sr. Kathryn Easley, OSB, Prioress, Benedictine Sisters of the Sacred Heart, led her religious institute through a strategic planning and decision-making process years before it became necessary and avoided the problems experienced by many other religious institutes. Sr. Marilyn Kuzmickus, SSC, General Superior of the Sisters of St. Casimir, embodied great wisdom as she dealt positively with problems that would have crushed lesser leaders. Richard Young, President, St. John Detroit Riverview Hospital, inspired his organization to succeed against formidable barriers that have closed many inner-city hospitals.

David Hannan, President of South Shore Hospital, created a powerhouse health system with a combination of visionary leadership and a legendary ability to attract and retain talented physicians and executives. David has been a mentor, client, and great friend for nearly three decades.

What magnificent leaders they are. What a great privilege it has been to know them and to learn from them. My admiration for each of them is profound. My greatest hope for the future is that I have the opportunity to continue meeting such gifted healthcare leaders.

PART ONE

Five Keys to Consulting Success

CHAPTER ONE

Knowing When to Use Consultants

D ECIDING WHEN TO use a consultant is the first step in a successful consulting experience. Healthcare organization leaders who fail to make this vital decision correctly are destined to be disappointed. If they bring in consultants who are not needed, they waste their organizations' time and money. If they avoid bringing in a consultant when one is truly necessary, even more time and money may be wasted. The objective of this chapter is to help organization leaders decide when to use consultants. The preliminaries to that important decision are understanding consultants and understanding the organization.

UNDERSTAND THE CONSULTANT

What exactly is a consultant? What do they do? Answering these questions is central to making an informed decision about whether or not to use a consultant. Think of the captain of a great ocean liner as a chief executive officer. The captain has years of experience and commands numerous officers who in turn oversee the ship's operation. The ship functions like many large enterprises with a leader, management, and employees. At sea, the captain, officers, and crew are truly the masters of their enterprise. However, at the very beginning and end of each voyage, the ship's captain turns to an outside consultant for the immensely important task of guiding the ship to and from the shore.

Who is this consultant? The harbor pilot. Since the beginning of the era of large ocean-going ships, harbor pilots have joined the captain and crew to guide the ship away from the dock, through the harbor, and out to sea. At voyage end, the harbor pilot again joins the ship to navigate the approach to land, using special expertise to bring the ship safely into its berth.

The harbor pilot's expertise in bringing ships into and out of challenging harbors makes him a consultant in the purest sense of the word. The pilot joins his experience with that of the ship's company and together they begin and end voyages as a team. The captain is not incompetent because he needs a harbor pilot. He does not argue that the pilot's services cost too much. The ship's owners do not begrudge the presence of this consultant. In turn, the harbor pilot could not guide the ship across the sea. He does not believe his special knowledge qualifies him to run the ship at sea or to ensure its safety if it were to encounter an unexpected hurricane. The captain and the harbor pilot each have their own place in this ocean-going enterprise. The captain is the chief executive, responsible and accountable for the ship and its voyage. The harbor pilot is the consultant, applying his special expertise to ensure safe departures and arrivals. Neither the captain nor the pilot is more important than the other—both are necessary to secure the safe and efficient operation of the ship.

Healthcare chief executives and consultants can learn from this analogy. Chief executives are the masters of their enterprises, but occasions do arise when they need the special expertise of others. Consultants, like harbor pilots, can offer chief executives the benefits of their special knowledge. Then, like harbor pilots, consultants should take their leave. Too often, chief executives do not ask for help when they need it. Just as often, consultants do not depart after their assignment is completed. Both situations can lead to disappointment.

KEY STEPS TO DETERMINE IF CONSULTANTS ARE NEEDED

Consultants perform many useful services for healthcare organizations, but they should only be retained when their special expertise is needed. Healthcare leaders should use this expertise to better their organizations. Consider the following four steps to determine if a consultant is needed:

1. understand the organization;
2. identify the problem or opportunity;

3. articulate the desired outcome; and

4. evaluate consulting and non-consulting alternatives.

Understand the Organization

Leaders must first know their organization's strengths and weaknesses before they can determine whether they need a consultant. What resources does the organization have? Do senior executives or middle managers have the expertise needed to solve the problem or pursue the opportunity? If the expertise is available within the organization, can staff members be relieved of current responsibilities to focus on the problem or opportunity long enough to achieve the desired result?

A common mistake chief executives make when confronted with a critical problem or opportunity is to be too generous in their assessment of in-house expertise. Even if they realistically assess internal resources, chief executives frequently assume their staff can work miracles on the problem or opportunity while continuing to perform their ongoing responsibilities with excellence. Other chief executives overlook talent right under their noses in the rush to hire outside consultants to solve a problem or bring an opportunity to fruition.

Both extremes are harmful. Attacking a key problem with weak internal resources inevitably leads to further problems that prove more expensive and time consuming to solve than the original issue. Ignoring appropriate internal expertise leads to resentment by the very people who could have solved the problem in the first place, not to mention the unnecessary expense of hiring consultants who were not needed.

Understanding an organization also requires evaluating and acknowledging political realities surrounding both problems and opportunities. One such political reality is the fact that people sometimes listen and respond better to an outsider. A chief executive may resent this notion. Resentment, however, does not make this phenomenon any less real.

Another factor relevant to retaining a consultant is the sensitive question of whether the organization has the funds. Hiring consultants costs money. If the organization does not have enough money to hire the most capable consultant, it should do the best it can with internal resources. An organization should not look for an inexpensive, unqualified consultant or ask a highly qualified consultant to compromise his or her integrity to make an engagement affordable. Both organization and consultant will be disappointed with these compromises.

Perhaps the most implicit factor in understanding the organization is assessing whether or not it will have the resources and resolve to implement a solution. If staff cannot or will not implement the solution, regardless of whether a consultant is retained, the organization should not bother going through the problem solving or opportunity exercise.

Boardroom Makeover: A hospital chief executive considered hiring a consultant to help restructure the hospital's board of directors. The board was dysfunctional, spending most of its time on minutiae and delving into operational matters. The chief executive talked with several prominent governance consultants who offered proposals to overhaul his board. After reviewing the proposals, the chief executive concluded that he personally had the expertise to restructure the board.

This chief executive recognized that he was facing primarily a political problem. The problem lay not with a dysfunctional board, but a dysfunctional board chairman. He enlisted the help of several board members and successfully encouraged the chairman to retire from the board. Could a consultant have achieved this success? Probably not. This chief executive knew his organization. He acknowledged the problem and its political aspects. He then successfully solved the delicate problem with internal resources.

Identify the Problem or Opportunity

The ability to clearly identify and articulate a problem or opportunity is an important factor in the decision of whether to retain a consultant. Some problems are obvious, such as an unanticipated financial loss, malpractice suit, or failure to achieve full accreditation by Joint Commission on Accreditation of Healthcare Organizations. Similarly, some opportunities are also obvious, such as developing a strategic plan, building an outpatient facility, or creating a new clinical service to better serve the hospital's patients. The decision to use a consultant for such issues is straightforward. If the organization does not have the internal resources or time to address the issue, consultants are the answer.

But what if the problem or opportunity is not obvious? For example, what is a board to conclude when the organization's chief financial officer or chief nursing officer position is subject to constant turnover? What is a chief executive to conclude when the number of newborn deliveries declines every year while the community's population is growing and the hospital across town enjoys a thriving and growing obstetrics business? What can an operating room director conclude when she observes that the post-surgical infection rate for one orthopedic surgeon's patients is triple that of his colleagues?

These subtle problems and opportunities require something more than simple analysis. They require leaders to acknowledge potential shortcomings of their organization's people, systems, or facilities. The ability to identify internal weaknesses is critical to the decision to retain a consultant. Many organizations can identify the problem but are then incapable of acknowledging that the cause could be internal. Instead, they may go to great lengths to look for external causes.

The truth is many healthcare leaders cannot or will not admit their organization's shortcomings. They hire a consultant to look for causes beyond their organization's control rather than admitting that the problem is within the organization. On the other hand, healthcare leaders who carefully research and articulate their organizations' problems and opportunities are in the best possible position to judge whether a consultant is needed. If the consulting approach is then chosen, consultants can be effective in discerning solutions, as the following example illustrates.

> **Boardroom Revolt:** Over a ten-year period a hospital experienced turnover of its chief executive position every two years. Each chief executive officer was fired by the board. At each termination, the board retained an executive search consultant to start the chief executive recruitment process all over again. Four out of the five searches were performed by the same executive search firm. A new search consultant was retained for search number five.
>
> During the search, one candidate contacted each of the four preceding chief executives. He learned that board members were not honest about what they wanted in a chief executive and had not faced their many internal problems. Board members said they wanted a strong leader. However, they actually wanted a weak leader who would look the other way while board leaders exploited their positions on the board for personal gain through their various business enterprises. Further, the former chief executives indicated that the former executive search firm knew

exactly what was going on but failed to confront the board. The candidate shared what he learned with the new executive search consultant.

During his personal interview, the candidate confronted the board over the subject of conflict of interest. This predictably angered the cadre of board members who had preferential arrangements for their banking, legal, and insurance businesses. The confrontation, however, emboldened other board members who resented the preferential arrangements. The search consultant made it clear that board problems must be resolved before a chief executive selection could be accomplished. A board revolt followed, which resulted in the resignation of the "good old boys." The newly configured board hired the insightful candidate. He is now the longest-tenured chief executive in the hospital's recent history.

Articulate Desired Outcomes

After identifying and articulating the problem or opportunity, you must next define the desired outcome. This is an important responsibility of the organization before retaining a consultant. The clearer the desired outcome, the better the consultant can assist the organization.

Articulating the desired outcome requires honesty, which is often difficult because it involves enumerating the organization's shortcomings. Failure to be completely honest almost always guarantees a less than desirable outcome. If a patient fails to fully disclose symptoms to his or her physician, the physician cannot make a timely and accurate diagnosis. Similarly, leaders who fail to disclose organization weaknesses and shortcomings cannot gain the full benefit of consultants' or staffs' expertise.

It is also crucial for leaders to articulate a timeframe for the consultation. Failure to do so can needlessly extend a consultation or shorten it to the point of a superficial exercise. If the organization needs a problem resolved in 90 days it must disclose this expectation to the consultant. Based on experience, the consultant may assist the organization in extending or shortening the timetable. It is vital for both the organization and the consultant to agree on the timetable for completion before the engagement begins.

Another important consideration in defining desired outcomes is the organization's advance commitment to following through on the consultant's recommendations. Too often, precious time and money are consumed by a consulting project only to have the most important step, implementation, fail. When a consultant is retained, the organization must be prepared to implement recommended solutions. Otherwise, it is better not to start the consulting process in the first place.

> **Ignoring the Inevitable:** Following five years of successful growth, a long-term care organization's financial performance declined sharply. After the first year of the downturn, the chief executive mollified the board, reassuring them that the next year would be better. When finances deteriorated for a second year, the board insisted on retaining a consulting firm to assess the situation.
>
> The consultant, jointly retained by the board and chief executive, concluded that key factors of the downturn resulted from poor strategic decisions made by the chief executive and his failure to reverse or change those decisions. The board and chief executive vehemently disagreed with these findings and fired the consultant. Another disastrous year followed, and the organization ran out of cash and was forced to close. Had the board acted on the consultant's findings, it is possible the organization would have survived under new executive leadership by reversing previous ineffective strategic decisions.

Evaluate Consulting and Non-Consulting Alternatives

After identifying a consulting opportunity and articulating the desired outcome, you are in a position to decide whether consulting assistance is needed. Whenever possible, use internal resources instead of retaining consultants. Consultants, no matter how enlightened, usually disrupt the organization's routine and require expenditure of considerable financial resources.

Avoiding the use of consultants requires the presence of internal resources capable of resolving the problem or taking advantage of the opportunity. The organization needs to ask itself the following questions:

1. Do we have the talent?
2. Does the talent have the time to devote without compromising their usual assignments?

Healthcare organizations very often have the internal talent to solve problems and capitalize on opportunities. But if either of the two questions above is answered in the negative, consulting may be the best approach. However, leaders should not underestimate the power and effectiveness of a highly motivated individual or internal team of individuals who are given the opportunity to solve a problem. In fact, the mere consideration of hiring consultants can be an extraordinarily motivating factor for an organization's staff.

If consultants must be considered because of limited internal resources, executives need to ask themselves three further questions:

1. Can we find the best consultant?
2. Can we afford to retain the best consultant?
3. Are we willing to do what the consultant recommends?

A negative response to any of these three questions should prompt reconsideration. If the organization is not willing to spend the time or money to find the very best consultant, it should not bother looking. If the organization cannot afford the best, it should not settle for second best. And, most importantly, if the organization finds the best and can afford them, it should not proceed unless leadership is prepared to take the consultant's advice.

The decision whether to retain a consultant is not necessarily straightforward. It is quite reasonable to blend consulting with internal resources. If the organization has the in-house talent, but not the time, a consultant can supplement internal resources and get the problem solved working as part of a team. Some consulting firms are reluctant to participate in the blended approach because it has the potential to lessen control and reduce professional fees. However, it is the healthcare organization that should run the project. If a blended approach is best, the organization should seek out a consultant who embraces rather than resists this collaborative approach.

Pathway to Success: Hospital leaders and staff wanted their organization to become the region's preeminent facility for the care of stroke patients. They had excellent facilities, superb physicians, and dedicated nursing and rehabilitation professionals. However, they lacked a cohesive approach to treatment and cost effectiveness.

A team of administrators, physicians, nurses, and rehabilitation staff assembled to focus on this opportunity and challenge. They invented what they referred to as the 80/20 rule. The team believed the organization's staff had 80 percent of the capability to become the best but they needed 20 percent outside expertise to complement their skills. They sought a consultant with expertise in clinical pathways to contribute ideas to the team's plans.

Together the 80/20 team and the consultant succeeded brilliantly. They created an award-winning approach to stroke care and significantly reduced the cost of stroke care by lowering patient length of stay and promoting early return to the activities of daily living.

CALCULATE THE COST AND BENEFITS OF CONSULTING

It is extremely rare that an organization can precisely evaluate the cost and the benefit of a consulting engagement. In most instances, costs can be accurately determined by adding up the consultant's professional fees and expenses. All the expenses associated with a consulting engagement should be included. Some consultants fail to articulate the total expenses, and organization leaders sometimes fail to ask what they are. However, adding up the total cost of a consultation is usually a straightforward calculation.

Determining the benefits of a consulting engagement is much more elusive. How does a board calculate the benefit of removing an ineffective chief executive officer or an unscrupulous board chair? How do hospital leaders calculate the benefit of taking privileges away from a physician whose length of stay is excessive or whose infection rate is triple the national average? Often the benefit calculation becomes a subjective judgment that defies precise calculation. In those instances, it is useful to hypothesize what the situation and outcome would have been without intervention.

Visualize the dilemma created by a surgeon whose infection rate is too high. Can retaining a consultant create a specific, calculable benefit? Perhaps. It might be possible to project the costs of extended hospital stays, higher malpractice costs, and extra treatment and pharmaceutical resources dedicated to patients who have been operated on by the surgeon in question. However, at best, these calculations are imprecise estimates of the benefits of either changing the surgeon's techniques or revoking the surgeon's privileges.

On the other hand, can the hospital allow a problematic surgeon to continue to operate? No. Can it calculate the precise cost of allowing the surgeon to continue or the benefit of changing or removing the surgeon? No. Is revoking the surgeon's privileges the right thing to do for reasons of patient care? Yes. So the benefit may be viewed as worthwhile, regardless of the cost of making the necessary change.

Another consideration in the cost and benefit calculation is the "true" or long-term cost of a consulting initiative that fails. Costs may go far beyond the initial professional fees and expenses. Costs associated with staff turnover, retraining, and service declines may sometimes meet or exceed the cost of the original consultation, as indicated below.

> **Reengineering Disaster:** The administrators of a medical center retained a large and well-respected consulting firm to reengineer its patient care services. The medical center had determined that costs were too high and reengineering was needed. The consulting firm proposed a $1.2 million professional fee plus an additional $300,000 for expenses. The firm assembled a team of 15 consultants, and a timeframe of one year for the reengineering was agreed on by consultants and client.
>
> The consulting process became an unmitigated disaster for the medical center. The reengineering process so disrupted the daily operation of the nursing department that the vice president of nursing, 8 nurse managers, and nearly 50 professional nurses resigned. Recruitment fees to replace executives and managers, plus outside agency fees to replace the nurses who resigned, ran into the millions of dollars. The medical center also experienced a loss of revenue of over $1.5 million when it was forced to temporarily close several nursing units because of insufficient nursing staff. The reengineering process was despised by physicians and patients alike. Eventually, the chief executive was fired because of the results of this failed consulting process. The only winner was the consulting firm, whose reengineering team moved on to the next client, either unaware of or uninterested in the devastation it left behind.

Tips on Avoiding Situations Destined to Fail

Even with the best intentions, some consulting situations are destined to fail. Sometimes consultants bear the responsibility for failure. All too frequently, healthcare leaders themselves are to blame. In other circumstances, both organizations and their consultants fail together. The following tips can help healthcare leaders and consultants succeed with their mutual endeavors.

Use Consultants Appropriately

Consultants cannot solve every problem or pursue every opportunity faced by healthcare leaders. Organization leaders can resolve many situations if they have the insight, resources, and necessary fortitude to make changes. Decisions about how to handle ineffective managers or passive/aggressive medical staff leaders do not require consultants. These decisions require organization leaders to do their jobs. Consultants can never substitute for a leader who abdicates his or her management responsibilities.

Pay for Quality

Executives who truly need consultants can be their own worst enemies when it is time to retain outside help. Sometimes an organization seeks out not the best consultants, but the least expensive. To ensure success, the organization must hire the best consultant for a particular problem or opportunity and be prepared to pay for quality advice. Obtaining inexpensive advice often limits the results to superficial solutions and ineffective outcomes. Of course, a high price tag on consulting advice does not guarantee great results. The consultant must have the appropriate skills and experience and the organization's leaders must support the consultant to achieve the best results.

Establish Goals and a Timeframe

Goals should be clearly established for all consultations and a timeframe determined for beginning and ending the consultation before it starts. It takes discipline to articulate goals before the consultation begins, but doing so helps both consultant and organization achieve them within a desired timeframe.

Maintain a Positive Attitude

Leaders can doom a consulting engagement to fail by their own poor attitudes. If leaders view consultants negatively, the effectiveness of any consultant, no matter how talented, will be diminished. Snide references to "high-priced outsiders" undercut the consultants attempting to help the organization. In some cases, this attitude can be so destructive it compromises the consultant's ability to provide effective assistance.

Make It a Team Effort

Organization leaders must be willing to devote the necessary time to ensure consultation is a team effort between the organization and its consultants. Some leaders hire a consultant and then wait for weeks or months for a magic solution to appear. Little or no participation by the organization itself leads to failure. Only by working as a team and carefully monitoring progress throughout the consultation can an organization and its consultants achieve the most desirable results.

Implement

Implementation is the culmination of a successful consultation. Failure to implement wastes time and money. Whose fault is that? While some consultants may indeed do poor work, failure to implement a well-conceived recommendation rests squarely with the organization and its leadership.

Good Consulting Outcomes Require Good Clients

Good clients attract the best consultants. Further, they stimulate consultants to do their very best work. Some healthcare executives have blind faith in their own capabilities and fail to retain consultants even when this could yield a positive outcome. Just as detrimental is blind faith in consultants. An organization cannot delegate a problem to a consultant and then assume the consultant will have the complete answer. The synergy between an informed client organization and a capable and motivated consultant can be extraordinarily powerful.

What makes a good client? Consultants want to work with organizations that truly know their internal strengths and weaknesses. If a chief executive with this knowledge of his organization has decided that consulting resources are necessary, the consultant can be confident that the decision to retain him or her was based on a realistic conclusion that internal resources were not present or sufficiently available to solve the problem.

Another aspect of a good client organization is the ability to clearly articulate the problem or opportunity that makes the consulting engagement necessary. Consultants are most effective when they know with precision what outcomes are expected. Articulating the timeframe for achieving the outcomes is also critical. A good client knows what is wanted and when.

A team culture is another highly desirable attribute in a client. An organization that views consultants as extensions of their own resources rather than interlopers is more likely to succeed than an organization that views consultants as necessary evils to be tolerated rather than embraced for their skills. Working together, an organization and its consultants can achieve dramatic results, as shown in the following example.

Best of Both Worlds: A rural medical center faced a period of declining profitability after years of stellar performance. The highly respected chief executive decided that consulting expertise was needed. He did not want the "slash and burn" approach to cost reduction so common in the healthcare industry. Instead, he mobilized physician and management leaders and articulated the challenge. Improved profitability was vital to achieving future strategic plans. He expressed confidence in the organization's staff while pointing out that some outside perspectives could be useful in challenging leaders to learn from the experience of others.

A small consulting team known for their collaborative approach to financial performance improvement was retained. Together, internal leaders and consultants examined every conceivable revenue enhancement opportunity and cost-reduction idea. Employees and physicians were engaged in the process, making it a truly collaborative approach.

The outcome was dramatic: a $7 million improvement in the bottom line. The medical center's leaders viewed this result as their own accomplishment, as they well should have. The consultants provided low-key advice and challenged the medical center's staff, but the ideas to increase revenue and reduce costs truly came from within the organization. A great client and an effective consulting team together achieved dramatic results.

CONCLUSION

Organization leaders should do their best to resolve problems or capitalize on opportunities with internal resources. If they constantly need outside consultants, the problem may lie with themselves and their inability to do the job. If and when situations arise where consultants are necessary, organization leaders must clearly articulate the problem or opportunity and the desired outcomes to be achieved with the assistance of consultants. The leaders then must explore consultant options with the objective of retaining the very best advisors to meet the organization's needs and be prepared to pay appropriately for excellent consultants.

Once retained, consultants and organization leaders must become an effective team, creating a solution and implementing it to achieve the desired outcome. Good clients attract good consultants, whereas bad clients cannot be helped, even by the best consultants. The client ultimately controls the outcome. If leaders do not do their jobs well, consultants cannot make up the deficit. The next chapter explores techniques for selecting the best consultant to meet your organization's needs.

CHAPTER TWO

Selecting the Best Consultant

HEALTHCARE ORGANIZATION LEADERS generally do not do an adequate job of retaining consultants. They often wait too long to make the decision to hire a consultant and then do a superficial job of selection. Ultimately, they waste time and money on a hastily hired consultant. Selecting the best consultants to meet a healthcare organization's needs takes quality time and quality effort.

In selecting a consultant, you should thoughtfully evaluate good alternatives and retain the individual or firm that best meets your organization's needs. The operative word is "thoughtfully" because it implies a certain amount of due diligence on the part of the healthcare organization's leaders. Unfortunately, selecting a consultant is often a cursory decision or a decision made during a state of panic when a catastrophic problem has developed and the organization wants someone to solve it.

Excellent consultants, like excellent chief executives, are rare. Fortunately, excellent healthcare consultants are available in many different-sized firms, from solo practices to billion-dollar consulting enterprises. Selecting the right consultant for a particular problem or opportunity begins with organization leaders asking themselves enough questions to define the scope of work the organization needs performed and the type of expertise required to perform that work.

Excellent consultants, regardless of the size of their firm, have several attributes in common. They are creative. They are good communicators. They have excellent collaboration skills and form excellent relationships with clients. Of course, excellent consultants also have technical and process expertise in their chosen fields. The very best consultants have the rare ability to be completely honest and candid while motivating clients to change and implement even the most difficult strategies and solutions to problems. Complete honesty and integrity are the most valuable, yet rarest, attributes of any healthcare consultant.

Selecting the right consultant also entails getting good value for the investment in consulting fees. This can be best achieved if the organization establishes a value for the work to be performed before the selection process gets started. While it is true in consulting that you get what you pay for, organization leaders should decide in advance what a particular engagement is worth, and then seek out consultants who can deliver excellent results within that value range.

Selecting the consultant who best meets your organization's needs involves hard work. A superficial or panicked selection will always lead to a disappointing result. Due diligence in the selection process is the key to success.

RANGE OF CONSULTANTS AND FIRMS

Although there is infinite variation, consulting firms may be grouped into three categories: small, medium, and large. Small firms range from solo practitioners up to five consultants. Medium-size firms range from 6 to 50 consultants. Large firms employ more than 50 consultants. In healthcare, large firms have been dominated by the "bigs"—ten years ago it was the "big eight" accounting firms with healthcare consulting divisions, then the "big six," and more recently the "big five." Fallout from the Enron debacle may lead to another reduction in firms to the "big four." Several large general management consulting firms with divisions serving the healthcare industry also exist.

Positive aspects of the large firms are the depth and scope of professional expertise; the wide scope of resources; multiple domestic and international office locations; and high-quality, talented consultants, especially at the partner level. The downside of a large firm centers on the leverage system, which promotes the most talented consultants to partners who supervise less-experienced consultants rather than directly providing consulting services. The financial reward system for partners in large firms is often oriented toward supervising engagements rather than performing engagements. Other drawbacks to the large firms are high overhead, the constant emphasis on selling new consulting work, and professional staff turnover at all levels.

> **Big Shuffle:** A healthcare chief executive wished to retain a consultant to improve the performance of his organization's business office. After conferring with colleagues, he learned that one of the "bigs" had experience in that area. He further learned that the partner with the best reputation was located in the Los Angeles office, over 2,000 miles away. Although his hospital was located in the Midwest, he contacted the L.A. partner directly to inquire about his firm's business office services. The L.A. partner politely referred him to the Cleveland office partner.
>
> The Cleveland partner assembled a proposal literally overnight. The chief executive noted that the proposal specified staff consultants from several Midwest locations, but no involvement from the L.A. office. When the chief executive inquired, he was told that the L.A. partner could be the "engagement leader." Satisfied that he was getting the best team, the chief executive retained the big firm.
>
> During the course of the engagement, the chief executive had the opportunity to meet the L.A. partner only once. The engagement was only partially successful, and the chief executive concluded that while the consulting firm had a great reputation, the Midwest consulting staff was weak. He concluded that even with big firms, you must hire the consultant, not the firm, in order to achieve desired results.

Medium-size healthcare consulting firms tend to focus on a particular aspect of consulting, such as facilities design, financial planning, or marketing strategy. Generally, medium-size firms have evolved from successful small firms. Positive aspects of medium-size firms are that they have focused expertise and high-quality consultants. Medium-size firms usually have enough resources to give personalized services to their clients. Drawbacks to medium-size firms can arise if they are growing quickly. Some growing firms hire new consultants who are not of the same caliber as the firm's founders. It is also sometimes difficult for client organizations to gain access to the successful partners of medium-size firms when they are expanding rapidly.

Small firms are usually small either because they choose to be small or because they are not successful enough to grow. Some solo practitioners and small firms have made a strategic choice to remain small to differentiate themselves from larger firms. Such firms are generally mature, with five or more years' consulting experience. Other small firms are simply not very good and have not grown because of their lack of success. Small firms and solo practices are often started by executives who leave management positions—sometimes by choice, sometimes not—and then go back into the field in a different capacity (most of these firms fail during the first five years). The advantages of a small firm can be excellent client service and focused expertise. Small firms usually have lower overhead, though not necessarily lower fees. Negative aspects of small firms include lack of depth and a tendency to be over- or underextended at any one point in time.

The question of determining what kind of consultant is best goes far beyond selecting the size of the firm. Determining who is the best consultant requires some initial soul searching by the prospective client organization's leaders.

DETERMINING WHICH CONSULTANT OR FIRM CAN BEST MEET THE ORGANIZATION'S NEEDS

Before retaining a consultant, you should first look within your own organization. An internal examination can provide a good framework for the consultant selection process. Initially, an organization's leaders need to ask themselves if the challenge needs a single advisor or a team of consultants with multiple skills. If you need advice on restructuring your governing board, a single experienced advisor might be appropriate. If you want to improve the flow of outpatient services, a team of advisors might be more effective.

The next question is whether the challenge is of a technical or process nature. If the challenge is technical, such as selecting the best new magnetic resonance imager (MRI), technical expertise is obviously needed. If, on the other hand, the challenge is to improve the quality of care to stroke patients, a process-oriented consultant might be the best choice. Your organization's culture and leadership style are also important considerations in selecting a consultant. Is a provocative consultant needed to shake up the organization? And is your organization mature enough to be shaken up without falling to pieces? Or is a more collegial consulting approach a better fit for your culture?

Timeframe is yet another consideration. Do you need lightning-fast results? Is the problem so severe that massive resources must be brought to bear as soon as possible? Is a slower timeframe more in keeping with your organization's needs? Some strategic planning consultants can complete the planning process in 90 days. They bring a team of consultants to an organization to conduct interviews, perform financial projections, study data, and discover strengths, weaknesses, and opportunities. After processing the data, the consulting firm is usually able to produce a credible report and recommendations for the future. An opposite approach is the strategic planning firm that takes six to nine months to work with the organization to produce a long-range plan, believing that processing time and discussion among the various constituencies is more important than speed in producing the final report.

Related to timeframe is consulting style. Do the consultants provide the answers or take the organization through the process for the organization to find its own answers? In the strategic planning example, fast consultants are providing answers. Slower consultants are facilitating the organization in finding answers on its own. Both methods have their place, depending on the needs of the organization. The important thing is for you to decide which approach is needed. Then the selection process for the best consultant to meet the desired objectives can begin.

A final question that the organization's leaders may ask themselves is what potential harm could be done to the organization by retaining certain consultants. It is amazing that healthcare chief executives honestly seeking to improve their organizations may hire a certain firm for turnaround or cost-reduction purposes, even though the firm may have a well-known track record of getting chief executives fired. At the very least, the organization's consultant selection decision should, like physicians, do no harm.

DETERMINING THE WORTH OF THE CONSULTATION

Determining the budget available for consulting is important. Organization leaders must decide what the consultation is worth to the organization. Defining a "value range" in advance is critical; otherwise, the consultants will determine the value in their proposal. The price, in the form of professional fees, may not correspond with the value of the engagement to the organization. For example, if the consulting firm is overextended, it may inflate professional fees to make the engagement worthwhile for them. If the firm has a specialty niche, it may inflate professional fees because of the lack of competition. And, if the client is desperate, as financial crisis turnaround clients normally are, the consulting firm may name an astronomical fee knowing full well the client has limited choices.

Although consulting fees for a particular engagement should not be the only consideration, they are an important consideration. All other things being equal, fees may be the determining factor in selecting a consultant. But "all other things" such as expertise, availability, references, and interviews are rarely equal. Special care must be taken to avoid selecting a consultant based on fees only. Consulting fees should be looked at as a good investment.

If your healthcare organization desires to improve its financial performance by one million dollars per year, what is the value of that achievement? How much should you expect to pay for that accomplishment? Ideally, you would figure out this financial challenge by yourself, thereby avoiding any consulting fees. But in reality, you may need consulting help to achieve this goal. To make a million-dollar improvement in its bottom line, you should be prepared to invest significantly, perhaps as much as 25 percent of the improvement. Who could question the investment wisdom of spending a quarter to get a dollar in real returns? On the other hand, how is the value of using a consultant to streamline the governance process determined? How much is that achievement worth? It is worth what the chief executive officer or board chair believes it is worth.

Economics Lesson: A community hospital was experiencing severe problems with a disruptive and impaired physician. Its chief executive contacted several consultants with expertise with problem physicians and discovered a wide variation in professional fees. One firm proposed a team "intervention" approach with very modest fees to help the hospital deal with the physician. Another firm proposed a one-on-one approach with a professional fee three times as high as the first proposal.

The chief executive selected the team approach, believing that the hospital was getting more for its money. The approach was a complete failure, and the physician's behavior worsened. The hospital then retained the second consultant who almost immediately pinpointed the problem and worked successfully to place the physician in a substance abuse rehabilitation program.

The two consulting approaches represented wide differences in professional fees. One was much higher and worked. The other approach cost less, but did not work. The chief executive learned a valuable consulting economics lesson from this experience.

Establishing a value range before the search begins for the consultant provides a reference point to evaluate proposals. Consultants may also ask an organization's leader in advance if he or she has a budget in mind. Most organizations fumble this question by saying they want to see what the proposals say. It would be far better for the organization's leader to specify the range of value in advance. This way the consultant has the opportunity to tailor appropriate resources to meet the organization's investment range.

CREATING A "SHORT LIST" OF CONSULTANTS

After establishing what the organization is willing to invest, leaders should create a "short list" of three to five consultants to begin the evaluation process. Having more than five creates a tendency to be superficial in the selection process due to insufficient time to meaningfully evaluate consultant alternatives. Also, consulting firms may be wary of organizations entertaining large numbers of proposals because they believe these organizations are merely shopping for the best price. Paring the list of potential consultants down to five or less requires forethought and diligence. Alternatively, if the list contains only one or two consultants, why bother with due diligence at all? Creating a short list of three to five alternatives provides a balance of choice without expending too many resources.

Allow for diversity on the short list. Assuming the organization's leaders have asked themselves enough questions to determine what size consulting firm is best, the short list should contain some alternatives for evaluation. For example, if you determine that a large firm is optimal, you may want to consider three large firms along with one small and one medium-size firm. If a small firm is desired, the options could include three small firms along with a large and a medium-size firm. Diversity on the short list gives you the opportunity to consider alternative approaches offered by the other firms. Being exposed to different approaches may help refine the engagement scope to include items or ideas not previously considered or confirm the efficacy of the scope already defined.

How is a consultant short list developed? The best approach is to seek the advice and garner the experiences of trusted colleagues. If, for example, a consultant is needed to improve emergency room patient flow, the organization's chief executive should contact professional associates and question them about their experiences with emergency room consultants. If a colleague does not know any such consultants personally, he or she may know of another colleague whose opinion he or she respects who used the services of an excellent emergency room consultant.

Another excellent referral source is consultants who previously served the organization well. For example, if a past consultant has provided services to improve the hospital's operating room patient flow, he or she may know of professional colleagues with expertise in the emergency room. Consultants with past records of success are highly motivated to provide referrals that reflect positively on themselves and serve the client's interests well.

Attending conferences and professional education programs is another way to identify good consultants. The best consultants in any field are sought-after speakers. Attending a presentation is a good way to get to know the style and approach of a prospective consultant. Also, excellent consultants are often prolific writers of professional articles and books. Consultants with expertise who have also published can be an excellent source of prospective consultants. A simple Internet literature search can identify these potential prospects.

Consultant trade associations are a possible source of contacts, although not necessarily a guarantee of quality, as are state and regional healthcare associations. For example, the president of a state hospital association may have ideas on good executive search firms and can provide referrals to chief executives in the state who have recently used such firms.

When creating your short list, it is important to list consultants, not just consulting firms, especially when considering medium-size and large firms. For example, if a large firm has a good reputation in a particular area of expertise, it is vital to learn who specifically in the firm has produced good results. Unfortunately, the partner in one office may be a great consultant but the partner in another office may be mediocre. The short list should specifically name the partner or practice leader to contact. If that person is unavailable because of geographic territory considerations, you should keep looking.

After the short list has been created, it is a good idea to contact each of the firms to determine their potential interest and availability for the upcoming engagement. When three to five qualified consultants are interested, it is time to prepare the request for proposal (RFP).

USING THE RFP EFFECTIVELY

Requests for proposals provide a disciplined framework to select the best consultant. Organizations that forego this process miss an opportunity to evaluate the strengths and weaknesses of alternative consultants before retaining one. Chief executives often view the selection of a consultant as an informal process whereby they orally describe their problem or challenge to a few consultants and request an informal proposal to deal with it. This informality usually does not provide the consultant with sufficient information to prepare a quality proposal for the client.

Sometimes chief executives decide in advance who they will select and use an informal approach to produce a few quick competitive proposals. This is essentially dishonest, and many consulting firms no longer respond to such informal requests because they suspect that the selection decision has already been made.

RFPS require forethought. The process of writing a good RFP forces the organization's leaders to carefully consider what kind of help they need and how the selection decision will be made. Sample RFPs for specific kinds of consultants are discussed later in this book. An outline of a thorough RFP, which can be adapted to any type of consulting need, follows. A sample RFP using the following basic format is also provided in Appendix A.

The Basics of an RFP

Organization Background

The objective of this section is to describe the organization in a few concise paragraphs. The description should include a brief history, scope of services, special capabilities, governance structure, employment and professional staff overview, annual budget, and leadership background.

Problem or Challenge Background

This section is the organization's opportunity to concisely explain why a consultant is needed and to describe the problem to be solved or the challenge to be met. It is helpful to provide a brief history of the problem or challenge, including internal or consulting efforts to date.

Objective of the Engagement

The purpose of this section is to describe the organization's objectives during and after a successful consultation. It articulates the outcome the client desires to achieve and should be specific enough for the consultant to determine the deliverables for the engagement.

Scope and Timeframe

This section describes the desired work the consulting firm will perform, the overall process to be used, and the organization's available resources. It also specifies the timeframe for the engagement, including start and completion dates.

Deliverables

This section specifically describes what deliverables are expected from the consultant, including reports, presentations, schedules, and so forth. In essence, this section should define the successful fulfillment of the engagement.

Proposal Submission Expectations

This section specifies a submission deadline, the format for the proposals, the number of copies needed, a contact person who can provide additional information, if needed, and who will receive the completed proposals.

Selection Criteria

In this section, the organization articulates the criteria that will be used to select the consulting firm. The organization should specify the timeframe for consultant selection, including when interviews will be scheduled after evaluating the RFP responses.

Proposal Submission Expectations

In addition to describing their approach to the engagement, the consulting firm should provide the following information.

Qualification of the Firm

The consultants should have an opportunity to describe their approach to the organization's specific problem or challenge and the firm's experience in successfully completing engagements of this nature. A brief history of the consulting firm is also helpful in this section.

Qualifications of the Consultants

The consulting firm should identify the specific individual who will be assigned to the client and his or her specific expertise in completing the engagement. Special emphasis should be placed on the qualifications of the engagement leader. This section should also specify the number of references to be provided. Three to five references should be provided for each proposal. A few of these references should be at least a year or two old so the organization can learn how well the engagement went after implementation results became apparent. Finally, any potential conflicts of interest of either the firm or an individual consultant should be disclosed in this section.

Professional Fees and Expenses

The consultants should specify their professional fees, any associated expenses, and the desired payment schedule for the engagement.

When the RFP has been completed, it should be sent to the "short list" consultants for consideration. Care should be taken to schedule the release of RFPS so sufficient time is available to analyze the responses of the consulting firms. The typical amount of time needed to complete each stage would be:

- two weeks to develop the "short list";
- two weeks to prepare and release the RFP;
- three weeks for consultants to submit RFP responses;
- one week for the organization to analyze RFP responses and select finalists;
- one week to make reference checks on finalists; and
- one week to interview the finalists and select a consultant.

Ten weeks may seem like a long timeframe, but this schedule assumes that the organization leader hiring the consultant has many pressing duties and selecting a consultant must take place while performing his or her other daily tasks.

THE IMPORTANCE OF THOROUGH REFERENCE CHECKS

RFP responses and reference checks should assist the organization in narrowing the selection to a few excellent finalists. A minimum of two finalists should be evaluated for any important consulting engagement. References are the best way to evaluate how well consultants perform. Personal interviews are also important and should be performed after reference checks have narrowed the selection.

The consultants' RFP responses should provide at least three references. Ideally, the organization's leaders should personally contact all the references of the firms that submitted the best RFP responses. While time consuming, there is no better way to determine who can best serve your needs than asking former clients how well each consultant performed.

Checking recent references is important, but it does not provide a complete picture. One or two references from engagements that were completed at least a year or two prior to the proposed engagement should also be checked. This is especially important with certain kinds of consulting such as cost reduction, turnaround consulting, and executive searches, to determine the longer-term results.

Prospective clients should be very wary of consultants who cannot provide references further back than a year or two. If they fail to provide such references, perhaps it is because none of their clients survived the consulting engagement. Certain consultants acquire a well-deserved reputation for getting their clients fired, regardless of how well leadership was performing. They should be avoided.

> **Invincible Chief Executive:** A healthcare organization was in big trouble. Mounting financial losses, declining morale, and uncertainty about the organization's survival weighed heavily on the chief executive. He decided to retain a turnaround consulting firm to help him restructure the organization. Several prominent firms were interviewed, and he asked the one he preferred for references from recent assignments. None were provided. The firm explained that its work was highly confidential, and it could not provide names of former clients.
>
> The chief executive had heard rumors that although this firm was very good, chief executives sometimes lost their jobs during a turnaround they orchestrated. He acknowledged this reputation, but concluded he was so capable that he could "handle" the turnaround consultants. He retained them and was fired four weeks later, joining the "confidential" client list of this high-profile turnaround firm.

Reference calls need not be lengthy or burdensome. Key questions for any consultant reference check should include:

- What was the scope of the consultant's work?
- Did the engagement meet your expectations?
- What were the best and worst aspects of working with the consultant?
- Was the engagement completed on time and within the agreed-upon budget?
- Was the value of the work to your organization equal or greater than the professional fee?
- Have the results of the engagement fulfilled long-term expectations?
- Would you hire this consultant again?
- Is there someone better that you could recommend?

Reference checking is a very enlightening process. Past clients are generally very willing to share their consulting experiences with other organizations. Their feedback, along with the RFP responses, should enable any organization to enter into the final selection process well informed and ready to make an excellent decision.

SELECTING THE BEST CONSULTANT AND NEGOTIATING PROFESSIONAL FEES

The final step in the selection process is personal interviews. If you started with five potential consultants, RFP responses and reference checks should narrow the choices to the best two or three as finalists. Organization leaders should schedule interviews to personally meet the consultants who will perform the work. It is best to avoid "beauty contest interviews" where consultants are kept waiting in a hallway while other consultants are interviewed one at a time for twenty minutes each.

Consultant interviews should be handled with the same courtesy and dignity as hiring a key executive. This is an opportunity for an organization to get to know a consultant and for a consultant to get to know a prospective client. During the interview, the consultant's answers to the following questions can be enlightening.

- What is your consulting style and why has it been successful?
- Why is your approach or your firm's approach more successful than your competitors'?
- How much of your consulting practice is based on repeat clients or referrals from former clients?
- What was your least successful engagement and what did you learn from it?
- How do you deal with a poor attitude toward consultants?
- How are you going to help my organization be successful with this engagement?

Care should be taken to introduce the consultant to key members of the organization who will work closely with him or her. Immediately following the interviews, the organization's leaders should ask themselves these four important questions:

1. Do we believe the consultant can do the job successfully?
2. Is the consultant compatible with our organization and us?

3. Will the consultant always be truthful with us, or will he or she be politically correct?
4. Do we really want to work with this consultant?

Interviews are opportunities to determine if the appropriate chemistry exists between consultant and organization. If the organization's leaders have written a good RFP and conducted thorough reference checks, it can be safely assumed that the consultant finalists under consideration are qualified. The purpose of the interview is to help the organization decide whom they want to work with one on one. When that decision is made, it is time to finalize the all-important matter of fees.

Fees have not yet been mentioned as a selection factor. Although some would consider this the deciding factor, the consultant should be selected based on quality factors, not just professional fees. Once it has been determined which consultant is the first choice, organization leaders and the consultant should finalize the matter of professional fees. If the firm is significantly more expensive than alternatives, the consultant of choice should be given the opportunity to revisit the proposed fee. Perhaps the consultant could adjust the fee or the client could consider changes in the scope of the engagement to make lower fees feasible.

Working together, the prospective client and the consultant of choice can reach a win-win decision on fees if they are both flexible. This is a good test of their ability to work successfully together. If an agreement is reached, the engagement can begin with both parties feeling like winners. If agreement cannot be reached on fees, the organization leaders should move on to their second choice. True bargains rarely exist in consulting. An organization trying to skimp on consulting fees will find itself hiring a cheap consulting firm and getting cheap work in return.

With the selection process concluded, one last step remains. A contract or letter of engagement should be completed and signed. Well-crafted RFPs become the basis of well-drawn consulting contracts. A sample letter of engagement that can be adapted to various consultations to governing boards, management, and clinical staffs is provided in Appendix B.

CONCLUSION

There are no shortcuts to making a good consultant selection. Organization leaders must think through their needs and articulate their expectations in a well-conceived RFP. To succeed, an organization must evaluate the RFP responses carefully, check references thoroughly, interview effectively, and make the final selection among the best-qualified consultants for the assignment. Such diligence will be rewarded with a thoughtful selection and the creation of mutual respect between client and consultant, which leads to a successful engagement. Once the selection is made, the next challenge is working effectively with the consultant to achieve the organization's desired goals.

CHAPTER THREE

Working Effectively with Consultants

IRING A GOOD CONSULTANT does not ensure positive results. Healthcare leaders often spend too little time working with the consultants they retain. Like the hiring process, working effectively with consultants takes quality time. If more organization leaders spent quality time on their projects after consultants were hired, they would receive better results. A consulting engagement is only as good as the organization's leaders make it.

Consulting is an investment. When an organization retains consultants, it expends financial and personnel resources. Consultants may be deployed to help the organization solve an acute problem or help it take full advantage of an opportunity. In both instances, consultants may help the organization considerably, or may be a complete waste of time and money. The difference in outcomes depends on how effectively the organization works with consultants, which is, ultimately, the responsibility of organization leaders. Capable leaders who strive to collaborate effectively with their consultants are rewarded with excellent results. Weak or ineffective leaders typically believe they can delegate their organization's problems to consultants—and they are always disappointed with the results.

Advance planning and good communication throughout the engagement is sure to pay excellent dividends for the organization. Organizations that emphasize planning and communication receive high value for their consulting investments. Thorough preparation ensures that the consultants will strive to do their best work, thereby achieving organization objectives. Creating an environment of mutual respect between the organization and the consultant also pays dividends. The organization that welcomes consultants as members of the leadership team can expect to receive the very best effort.

INTRODUCING CONSULTANTS TO YOUR ORGANIZATION

Success begins with good introductions. Introducing consultants to your organization actually begins during the pre-engagement interview process. If the organization involves key leaders in the consultant selection process, those leaders will already be familiar with the consultants. After selection, it is very important for leadership to positively introduce the consultants to the rest of the organization.

The chief executive or senior executive responsible for the engagement should announce the consultant selection at key meetings and by written communication to all staff who will be working with the consultants. These announcements should stress the need and purpose for retaining the consultants, background of the consultants, and the objectives the organization wishes to achieve with the help of the consultants. A timetable for the consultants' presence should also be communicated in the initial announcement.

When consultants arrive to begin work, they should be personally introduced to the organization's staff, including support staff. The consultants should meet with the secretarial staff with whom they will be working and provide background on the assignment and contact information for when they are not present within the organization. This extra effort and courtesy will help both the consultants and the organization throughout the engagement.

During the time consultants are present in the organization, they should be invited to attend key organization meetings as guests, even if the consulting assignment does not affect that particular aspect of the organization. For example, if a consulting team was working with senior management to address an operations problem in the emergency room, it would be advisable to introduce the consultants at the organization's next management meeting and allow department managers to ask questions about the assignment and inquire about rumors that may be generated by the consultants' presence.

Consultants always seem to be the subject of an organization's rumor mill. In an information vacuum, staff will always assume the worst. If the consultants are charged with helping reduce patient waiting time in the emergency room, the rumor mill may quickly broadcast that the consultants were really hired to get rid of 20 percent of the nursing staff. The only effective way to counteract the rumor mill is to communicate fully and honestly within the organization about the consultants' presence.

In addition to rumors, the presence of consultants seems to frequently bring out the most negative people within the organization. Without sufficient communication, an organization can usually count on a vocal and passionate critique of the consultants, regardless of their assignment. "They are too expensive ... they don't know any more than we do ... they're too young ... they don't know how unique we are" are all common refrains. Consultant bashing is a frequent and damaging behavior in organizations that do not make the time and effort to properly introduce their consultants.

COMMUNICATION THROUGHOUT THE ENGAGEMENT

Good communication can make even the most challenging consulting assignment proceed more smoothly. It begins with introducing the consultants to the organization's staff in a positive manner and establishing an engagement calendar. Good communication affects every aspect of the entire engagement.

Every organization has certain unique characteristics and perspectives and leaders should brief consultants about actions that may compromise their ultimate effectiveness. Most organization leaders have had both good and bad experiences with consultants. The cumulative bad experiences can be characterized as self-destructive behaviors for new consultants. For example, if consultants stay in the luxury hotel one block from the organization during a turnaround engagement instead of the more moderately priced hotel four blocks away, they may inadvertently discredit themselves in the eyes of the organization's leaders and staff. Every organization leader knows these sensitive behaviors and should warn their consultants about them before their effectiveness is compromised.

Once a consulting engagement has been initiated, it is very important to schedule sufficient time to allow the consultants to brief the client about progress, inevitable problems, and adjustments. These periodic briefings often fail to occur or are only superficial in nature. It takes discipline for the consultants to insist on these periodic updates and discipline on the part of the organization to make sufficient time available for the briefings.

Probably the most important aspect of communication throughout any consulting engagement is honesty. Consultants should be absolutely committed to providing honest feedback to the client. Honesty can be very difficult at times, since it can cause embarrassment or even anger on the part of organization leaders. But organizations hire consultants for their objectivity, and consultants are obligated to provide it, even if clients occasionally react in a defensive manner.

Organizations have an obligation to be honest, too. Sometimes leaders wait for their consultants to "discover" the truth, perhaps as some kind of test. This behavior is effectively game playing with the consultants. Organizations should provide all relevant information to their consultants, even if it is embarrassing. To do otherwise is to risk not getting the full value and benefit of the consultation. Mutual honesty is essential to achieve objectives and ensure the creative process between organization and consultant is maximized.

IMPORTANCE OF SCHEDULING AND CALENDAR PLANNING

The start of any consulting engagement is the optimum time to plan the schedule and calendar of meetings for the entire engagement. Major milestones, such as the date of completion, are agreed upon before beginning the engagement. Although it requires great discipline on behalf of both the consultants and the organization, planning the meetings and key milestones to attain the major goal should be undertaken as one of the first priorities.

The engagement calendar should be planned with the organization's leaders and consulting team and should include all key meetings, interviews, presentations, and report deadlines throughout the engagement. It is very beneficial for organization leaders to examine their calendar of regularly scheduled meetings such as board meetings, management meetings, and clinical staff meetings. Such meetings are an excellent opportunity for consultants to provide periodic status reports during the engagement.

It is vital for the consultants to specify all required client meetings so they can be scheduled on the appropriate staff members' calendars immediately. Healthcare organizations are busy enterprises led by busy people. It is extremely helpful for all the leaders to know what is required of them throughout the consulting engagement. Although additional meetings may become necessary, most meetings can be scheduled in advance.

Once the engagement calendar is set, it is necessary for the consultants and the organization to stick to it. Emergencies may come up within the organization or for the consultants, but consultants and organizations should adhere to the engagement calendar and make as few changes as possible. Last-minute scheduling of important meetings may cause resentment. A carefully planned calendar is one of the best ways to show respect for each other's time.

GETTING THE RIGHT PEOPLE INVOLVED WITH THE CONSULTANTS

The success of any consultation depends on getting the right organization leaders involved. Too often organizations hire consultants, breathe a sigh of relief, and wait for miracles to occur. They may believe that for all that money, consultants should walk on water, leap tall buildings in a single bound, and stop bullets with their bare hands, not to mention solve every last one of the organization's problems.

It is not so simple. Hiring consultants may begin the problem-solving process, but it most assuredly does not end it. The right people must be assigned to work with the consultants. Who are the right people? In some cases it is obvious. If a consultant is trying to help reduce the rate of post-surgical infection in the operating room, the operating room manager and chief of surgery must be involved. Staff from infection control and the laboratory are also obvious choices. But the consulting process may also benefit from the insights of surgeons, operating room nurses, housekeeping, and surgical unit support staff. Intensive care nurses and respiratory therapists may also have important insights. Anesthesiologists, pulmonologists, and internists may be able to offer suggestions and feedback valuable to the objective of reducing infections.

An internal team must be assembled to work with the consultants, regardless of the objective of the engagement. Every aspect of the problem should be considered when assembling this team. In addition, the attitudes of the team members must be considered. Individuals who harbor resentment toward consultants will be disruptive to the consulting process. Individuals with a poor attitude in general may not be constructive team members. Some organizations purposefully assign such people to consulting teams in the hopes the consultants can "straighten them out." It never happens. Problem employees should be dealt with by the organization's leaders, not its consultants.

Keeping the right people informed throughout the engagement is also very important. Periodically scheduled project meetings serve both as brainstorming sessions and to keep the staff informed.

GOOD ETIQUETTE LEADS TO EFFECTIVE TEAMWORK

It may seem counterintuitive to mention etiquette in the context of consulting, yet good manners go a long way toward ensuring a successful consultation. If organization staff demonstrates good etiquette toward consultants, it makes the job easier and the outcome more likely to be useful. If consultants demonstrate good behavior within the organization, they will be in a better position to work as an effective team with their client.

What constitutes good etiquette in a consulting engagement? It begins with providing suitable working space for consultants. It might be desirable to put a health department inspection team in the basement next to the boiler plant with broken-down furniture and only pay phone service, but it probably does not make sense to put the organization's strategic planning consultants in the same dismal location. A conference room or empty office with phone service is ideal and very much appreciated by most consultants. Access to fax machines, e-mail lines, and secretarial assistance are also helpful.

Temporary access to the organization's parking facilities and cafeteria also go a long way toward making the consultants feel important to the organization. Paying consulting bills on time is important, too. Most consultants dread having to act as a collection agency at the same time they are helping an organization solve an important problem.

One of the most important considerations an organization can give any consultant is to always be open and honest. If a problem develops during the engagement, the organization's leaders should communicate the problem so the consultants can resolve it to the client's satisfaction.

What about consultant etiquette? Consultants should always show proper respect for the client's property and facility. Office space should always be kept clean and organized and phone lines should not be abused. Consultants should never use fax lines, phones, or other facilities to do business other than the client's. Consultants should show proper respect for the organization's time by always arriving at meetings on time and never canceling or postponing meetings because of the needs of other clients. Canceling a meeting because of illness or a delayed flight is one thing; canceling to free up time to make a sales presentation elsewhere is quite another and shows a lack of respect.

> **Divided Loyalty:** A healthcare organization retained a financial consulting firm for help in planning for a future bond issue. Consultants assigned to the project made themselves right at home in a vacant office in the executive suite. In between meetings with the organization's leaders, they were phoning other current and prospective clients. A steady stream of faxes arrived daily from other clients at the consultants' temporary office. Draft reports were reviewed, proposals finalized, and problems were handled, all for other clients while the consultants were nominally working on the organization's problem.
>
> The chief executive was irritated that the consultants practically commandeered his assistant, who was more than irritated. The consultants' rude behavior continued throughout the several-month engagement, with the chief executive becoming more and more upset. When the engagement concluded, the chief executive vowed to never again use that consulting firm. Unfortunately, he never shared his reasons for his decision with the consultants. As a result, there is little doubt that other clients are being similarly abused.

Consultants must respect the chain of command of the organization for which they are working and keep the organization's leader in charge of the consulting engagement fully informed. Consultants should never criticize an organization when working with another client. And, perhaps the biggest etiquette issue of all, confidentiality must be maintained. A consultant must never share any information about the organization to anyone outside the organization before, during, or after the engagement. A consultant who violates confidentiality is committing a gross breach of etiquette and violating professional ethics.

Good etiquette is a necessity from both organization and the consultant. When present, the best work is accomplished. When absent, good work becomes difficult, if not impossible.

GETTING THE MOST FROM THE CREATIVE PROCESS

A consulting engagement ideally involves the best creative thinkers of the organization and the consultants. Even with the best intentions, there are usually significant barriers to the creative process. Organization leaders sometimes have preconceived notions about what will work and what will fail. Consultants, too, bring with them their own preconceived notions. How can barriers to creativity be overcome?

Every consulting situation, whether it is a problem to resolve or an opportunity to explore, has uniquely creative solutions. It is the synergy of ideas, or brainstorming, between organization and consultants that can produce such solutions. The best way to enhance the creative process is to acknowledge the expansive knowledge base of organization and consultants and generate new ideas by applying that knowledge in new ways. Generally, the organization has an understanding of what has been tried before and consultants know what has worked in similar situations. By combining this expertise and brainstorming without constraint, new solutions will emerge.

Involving all constituencies in the brainstorming process also yields good results. Consultants and organization leaders may be gifted with knowledge and creativity, but staff and physicians may contribute different ideas in the brainstorming process. Another important consideration is timing. Creativity is an evolutionary process. A singular flash of brilliance necessary to solve a particular problem does not often occur. Brainstorming ideas over several days, weeks, or even months can produce ideas that stand the test of critique and refinement. Organization leaders and consultants are well advised to let the creative process evolve over time, rather than expect a brilliant solution to emerge during a one-hour meeting.

Revelation in the Laboratory: A consulting team was engaged to help a community hospital reduce operating expenses. While the hospital was not financially distressed, the chief executive wanted to involve his administrative and department management staffs in brainstorming possible cost-reduction ideas. One aspect of the process involved carefully examining expenses in the laboratory department. Benchmark data indicated that some improvement was possible, but ideas to reduce costs were not readily apparent. The consultant pushed the laboratory manager for ideas.

The laboratory manager was resistant at first. However, she was persuaded to examine her systems, equipment, and staffing, and soon involved all of her employees in the brainstorming process. Over a period of weeks several ideas for reducing costs surfaced from these sessions. The consultant suggested the brainstorming, but did not dictate any particular cost-reduction approach. Ultimately, a 5 percent total reduction in the laboratory's budget was achieved through the creative efforts of the laboratory manager, physicians, and staff. In this instance, the creative solutions were present, and the consultant acted as a catalyst to bring them out in a manner that achieved results.

The "been there, done that" trap should be avoided in the creative process. Just because an idea failed two years previously does not mean that the time is not right to try it again. Just because an idea did not work with a past client does not mean it will not work with the current client. Creative solutions involve what works here and now. Rejecting ideas because of history is one sure way to kill creativity.

Creative synergy between organization and consultants is one of the greatest benefits of a consulting engagement. If organization leaders had all the answers, there would be no need for the consultants. On the other hand, if the consultants had all the answers, they could simply package the solution for easy implementation. Real-life problems rarely succumb to packaged approaches. Extracting the very best ideas from both consultants and clients can produce extraordinary synergy and successful solutions.

PLANNING FOR THE ENGAGEMENT'S CONCLUSION

Ideally, planning for the engagement's conclusion starts on the day it begins by establishing a firm completion date. Consulting should not be a never-ending process. It should have a distinct beginning and a distinct end.

The organization should achieve the desired outcomes by the conclusion of the consulting engagement. Rarely do organization leaders desire only a report of findings. They want actions or strategies to achieve their objectives. The conclusion should produce an action plan and implementation process, not an impressive-looking report. This is best achieved by a deliberative process and exchange of draft ideas near the end of the consulting engagement.

Consultants should verbally communicate their recommendations in draft form first. The client should thoroughly critique them, with the exchange resulting in changes and refinements to the recommendations. Following the oral presentation, the consultant should prepare a draft written report for further discussion and critique by the client.

Once the recommendations are agreed on, the final report can be prepared and submitted. By exposing the consultants' recommendations to both oral and written critiques, organization leaders have the opportunity to shape the final strategies and take ownership of the recommendations. An excellent consulting engagement is never just the sum of the consultants' expertise; rather it is the result of an intellectual exchange between organization leaders and consultants.

Communicating the findings is the next major step in successfully concluding a consulting engagement. Consultants may want to participate in communicating the findings to important constituencies within the organization. At other times the client must take the full responsibility for communication.

There is one last step in the process. Organization leaders should always meet with the consultants at the conclusion of the engagement and provide both positive and negative feedback to them. Excellent consultants welcome constructive criticism and will use it to improve the quality of their services to future clients.

CONCLUSION

Working effectively with consultants takes commitment, from both the organization and the consultants. Effectiveness does not happen automatically. Like respect, it is gained by careful attention to, and respect for, the organization's needs and the consultants' contributions. Failure to work effectively can lead to pitfalls that can ruin any consulting engagement.

CHAPTER FOUR

Avoiding the Common Pitfalls

Good intentions alone are not enough to achieve success in a consulting engagement. When consulting projects go wrong, it is usually because either the organization or the consultant makes a fundamental mistake. Most of these mistakes are avoidable. The first step in avoiding potential pitfalls in a consulting engagement is to understand what can go wrong.

Even when the reason for engaging a consultant is sound, the selection of the consultant is excellent, and the consultant and organization are poised to work well with each other, pitfalls can still derail a positive experience for either or both parties. It is not uncommon for organization leaders to have completely unrealistic expectations of what can be accomplished through the consultation. Alternately, consultants may not give the assignment their best effort and so doom the engagement to failure.

To achieve everyone's objectives, conscious effort must be made to identify the problems that can compromise a consulting engagement and to successfully overcome those problems. Avoiding or resolving potential problems will ensure success, whereas failure to recognize or prevent pitfalls always means someone will be disappointed during or at the end of the engagement. The objective of this chapter is to illustrate how to avoid the pitfalls that commonly befall healthcare organizations when consultants are retained.

HOPING FOR MIRACLES

For an organization, having either unrealistic expectations or waiting far too long to engage a consultant is a major pitfall. Consultants cannot perform miracles. In spite of their many excellent qualities, consultants can never compensate for a poorly led organization or one that will not face its own problems. If the organization is experiencing a major problem and that problem becomes a catastrophe, no consultant can arrive on the scene and magically make the problem disappear. First and foremost, leaders must know their organizations well enough—realistically acknowledging their internal strengths and weaknesses—to avoid working on a problem until it becomes a disaster. Not only is this poor management, but inevitably the solution will take longer and cost more.

Consultants are frequently asked to intervene after initially small problems become catastrophic. The entire turnaround consulting discipline thrives because organizations do not fix their problems before they spin out of control. Failures of the board, executive leaders, or medical staff cannot be remedied solely by consultants, even turnaround consultants. Good results in any consultation require organization leaders to recognize the problem, work hard, and apply discipline. Consultants can sometimes help resolve difficult challenges, but they should not be expected to clean up the messes of a leadership team that has failed to do its job properly.

DENYING REALITY

The opposite attitude to expecting consultants to perform miracles is to avoid retaining consultants at all costs. Countless organizations put off getting help until it is too late, at which point they are often willing to turn over responsibility and walk quietly away. Organizations experiencing financial distress are especially prone to put off getting help. Leaders in these organizations are adept at denying reality or unwilling to admit that they need help to return their organizations to financial stability.

Last Consultation: A community hospital experienced a rapid decline in financial performance. The chief executive was unwilling to acknowledge that the problems were within his control. He convinced his board that "everyone" was having trouble, and they believed him. After another year of rationalizing the decline, the hospital defaulted on a loan payment. Turnaround consultants were immediately hired by the board. The chief executive was fired and replaced, along with his entire administrative staff, by a team of turnaround consultants.

After six months of intensive turnaround efforts, and the expenditure of several million dollars in consulting fees, the hospital was sold to a nearby competitor. The consultants concluded it was too late to save the hundred-year old institution. Unfortunately, they had no miracle solutions. The only miracle was that the consultants got paid.

INSUFFICIENT RESOURCES TO ACHIEVE SUCCESS

Another pitfall that can lead to the failure of a consulting engagement is underestimating the resources needed to bring the engagement to a successful conclusion. Often, after an engagement is begun, it quickly becomes apparent that the problem or opportunity is far more complicated than either the organization or consultants anticipated. If the organization fails to respond by marshalling more resources, problems can quickly occur. At the same time, if the consultant fails to bring more resources to the situation, additional problems can arise.

Even when sufficient organization and consultant resources are appropriated, a timeframe that is too long or too short can derail the engagement. If the timeframe is too short, necessary research and consensus building may not take place to develop appropriate recommendations. Creativity takes time and cannot be rushed. On the other hand, if a too-long timeframe exists, the problem may worsen or turn into a completely different challenge. It is also difficult to sustain any consulting effort beyond a reasonable timeframe because the organization and consultants lose focus.

Planning Light: A medical center decided to create a new strategic plan. Several different consulting firms were evaluated before a firm that specialized in turnkey strategic planning was engaged. The firm possessed the capability to devote a large team of consultants that could do everything from background research to drafting strategic objectives with little input required from the client organization. The chief executive felt certain that this approach would yield an excellent strategic plan.

The chief executive wanted to complete the strategic plan in sixty days, in time for the medical center's fall board retreat. The short timeframe required the consulting firm to use far greater than the usual number of consultants, some of whom were quite inexperienced. Several teams of consultants arrived to begin work. After a hasty and superficial introduction by the chief executive, interviews began with the organization's leaders. The consultants diligently took notes and quickly discovered there were wide discrepancies among the various leaders in their ideas about the future strategic direction for the medical center.

Because of the abbreviated timeframe and the limited involvement of the medical center's leadership, the consultants drafted the strategic plan in somewhat of a vacuum. Based on their work for similar organizations, the consultants were confident, however, that their recommendations would meet with support. The chief executive agreed with the consultants' recommendations, and a strategic plan was prepared and delivered to the board several days before the fall retreat.

To say that the retreat was an extremely humbling experience for the chief executive and the consultants would be an understatement of considerable magnitude. Because there had been no time provided to discuss and refine the strategic recommendations, the board balked at accepting them. There was great debate during the retreat, not only about the recommendations, but also about the wisdom of the chief executive and the capability of the consultants. At the end of the retreat, the board directed the chief executive to start over, with a longer timeframe and a different consulting firm. The first process failed completely because of the lack of internal resources and, more importantly, the absence of enough time to refine and improve the strategic recommendations.

"UPSELLING" OF CONSULTING SERVICES

When organization leaders decide to retain a consultant, they should have a clear picture of what they want. It is the client's obligation to articulate what is needed from the consultant. The organization's leaders should avoid consultants who "upsell" when clients do not define clear expectations.

Upselling is a deceptive practice used by consultants to get organizations to purchase more of the consultants' services. It can occur at any point in an engagement, but is most likely to happen at the middle or end. Upselling occurs when the consulting firm working on one project tries to sell the client one or more additional services before the first engagement is completed. In most instances, purchasing additional services is deemed to be necessary before the original project can be completed. It is like buying a car and being told on delivery that the tires will be extra. The unwary client, or one that does not clearly understand and articulate the organization's needs, can become subject to upselling.

Upselling can also come in the form of creating new proposals for consulting services for areas unrelated to the original assignment. When consultants are retained to work on one project, they frequently are exposed to other problems or opportunities elsewhere in the organization. The pressure is so great on some consultants to sell additional work that they sometimes use the insider information they gain on one project to try to sell additional consultation work in other areas. Not only is this poor etiquette on the consultants' part, it may have the secondary effect of compromising the original project the consultants were retained to work on.

BAIT AND SWITCH STAFFING

When an organization retains a consultant, it expects to have the work performed by the people specified in the engagement agreement. It is not uncommon, however, for the organization's leaders to meet one consultant or team during the interview and proposal stage, only to find out that a completely different group will actually perform the work. Sophisticated organization leaders deal with this proactively by insisting on meeting, during the interview phase of the selection process, the actual people who will perform the consulting work. This is also an important point in a good contract or letter of agreement. Nevertheless, bait and switch problems persist.

In larger firms, it is common for a sales team to interact with the organization's leaders until the agreement is signed. Sales teams are usually excellent at selling, but do little, if any, actual consulting with clients. If organization leaders are not completely satisfied with the consultants' capability or their attitude when the engagement team begins work, they must insist on a change of personnel immediately. In obvious cases of bait and switch, in which the contracted team is replaced by substitutes, the engagement should be cancelled and new consultants hired.

In cases where a valid excuse is given for substitutions (such as illness, turnover, or personal emergency) organization leaders should evaluate the substitution. If not completely satisfied, the organization should insist on a change or terminate the engagement. The most common reasons for switching consultant teams usually do not bode well for the client. When a consulting team is switched to put the original team on a more lucrative engagement, that is unfavorable for the original client, not to mention unethical. A team switched because the original team is cleaning up another client's mess is also bad news for the original client.

> **Doctor Who:** An academic medical center needed a consultant to help improve physician quality in its anesthesia department. Several consulting firms that had physician expertise were interviewed and a very large firm was chosen to assist the medical center. The client's decision was based in large part on the physician presented by the consulting firm as the lead consultant for the engagement.
>
> When the engagement began, the physician leader was present, but was accompanied by another physician. The second physician was introduced as the principal consultant, and the original physician said that he would be overseeing the project. When the medical center's leaders objected to this new staffing arrangement, the consulting firm made it clear that the original physician was far too valuable to be involved in all the consulting work personally. His role was to supervise client assignments.
>
> The "supervising" physician was rarely seen during the four-month engagement. The principal consulting physician, although somewhat capable, did not have the skill of the original physician. The engagement ended with unsatisfactory results, and the medical center leaders vowed never again to be victims of bait and switch staffing schemes by consulting firms.

NEVER-ENDING ENGAGEMENT

Another common pitfall is that of the never-ending engagement. Sometimes the client organization is responsible for this pitfall. At other times, the consultants are the culprits. Whoever is at fault, this situation manifests itself when closure is not forthcoming on a consulting engagement.

When consultants are at fault, it almost always is related to the engagement's staffing. Consultants get pulled from one assignment to staff another. Not infrequently, turnover is a factor, especially with large consulting firms. If the agreed-on personnel are not available, the engagement often will not conclude on schedule. Upselling can be a significant cause of delay as well. If the engagement changes because new assignments are added, the original assignment suffers.

Consultants are not always at fault. Organizations can be the source of many delays. If the engagement calendar is not carefully crafted at the beginning of the engagement or adhered to in the midst of it, organization leaders are sometimes unable to give the consultants what they need. If meetings are not scheduled or they are endlessly delayed while secretaries try to merge busy consultant and organization leader calendars, the assignment lengthens. At other times, meetings take place on schedule but nothing productive happens. When consultants or clients become rigid in their ideas or strategies, stalemates occur.

Perhaps the most common cause for the never-ending engagement is reluctance by the organization to take action at the end of the engagement. If the engagement involves tough decisions or implementing challenging recommendations, it is not uncommon for organizations to delay endlessly. Consultants are reluctant to call attention to the delay in some cases, fearing retribution by the organization. It is rare that a delay, by either organization or consultants, results in a better outcome. Someone has to have the courage to say "Enough is enough." More often than not, it should be the consultant, but this is usually not one of a consultant's greatest strengths. That is how an organization ends up with an endless engagement.

Time to Go: A consultant had advised a healthcare organization for ten years. He had been instrumental in hiring the chief executive, appointing the board chair, and making numerous other important decisions during his time as a trusted advisor. However, after years of excellent relations, tension developed between the consultant and the board chair and chief executive. They disagreed on the strategic direction for the organization. The consultant held strong beliefs that the direction the organization was heading would lead to future problems. The board chair and chief executive were just as convinced that their approach was sound.

Escalating tension caused the consultant to step down despite the objections of the organization's leaders. He correctly concluded that he had overstayed his effectiveness and reluctantly gave up the organization as a client. The consultant knew that the organization had to find its own way in the future, as hard as that was to admit for both his ego and his checkbook. It was cold comfort several years later when the chief executive was fired, the board chair stepped down, and the organization nearly filed for bankruptcy.

BAD MANNERS YIELD BAD RESULTS

It may seem unusual or even odd to put so much emphasis on etiquette in the context of consulting. Just as healthcare administration leaders are not taught manners in business school, consulting firms do not teach good manners to their consultants either. In reality, however, manners have much to do with the outcome of consulting engagements.

If an organization behaves badly toward its consultants, it can be certain it will not receive the consultants' best work. Bad manners discourage initiative and divert attention from the assignment. Common sense suggests that if a consultant has two clients and one exhibits a positive attitude in all respects, that client will get the consultant's best efforts. The client who demonstrates a poor attitude will most certainly get a lesser effort. Just because the client is paying a fee does not ensure good work, especially in the presence of a poor attitude or bad manners.

On the other hand, consultants themselves are sometimes guilty of poor attitudes and bad manners toward the client. When a consultant fails to maintain confidentiality, for example, or abuses the trust the client places in him, the client will be discouraged to such an extent that the engagement objectives likely will not be achieved.

What can an organization do if the consultant demonstrates a poor attitude or bad manners? What is a consultant to do if the organization's leaders show a poor attitude toward the engagement? First, the parties should be honest about the effect of the behavior and try to work out their differences. If, however, they are unsuccessful, the right approach is to end the engagement. If a consultant is unable to get a client to show a properly polite attitude, he or she should quit. If the client is unable to have the consultant act in a similarly positive manner, the consultant should be fired. It takes courage for either party to take this dramatic step. To do otherwise, however, is a waste of time and money.

> **Bad Board Manners:** A consultant was retained to evaluate the governance structure of a large community hospital foundation. Trustee interviews revealed two distinct factions on the board. One faction wanted to modernize the governance structure and make changes in the officers who had been in place for over a decade. The other faction, currently running the board, wanted no changes. That faction went to great lengths to ostracize the consultant, both in private and during board meetings.
>
> The consultant talked to the leaders of both factions about his dissatisfaction with the trustees' attitudes. The leaders insisted that all trustees treat the consultant and the engagement with respect. After these discussions, things got worse. The trustees in power became more aggressively rude and disrespectful. As a result, the consultant terminated the engagement. A year later a boardroom coup took place, and the old regime was deposed. The consultant's recommendations were then reassessed and implemented. Termination of the engagement by the consultant was the precipitating factor in making the necessary governance changes.

MUTUAL DISSATISFACTION AT THE END OF THE ENGAGEMENT

No organization or consultant wants an engagement to end badly—unfortunately, however, it happens. A poor ending can usually be traced back to a poor beginning. If expectations are not made clear in the beginning, it is likely there will be problems at the end. If the engagement gets off to a poor start because of problems with the organization or consultant, it is likely the problems will get worse rather than better.

When an engagement ends poorly, the organization usually pays the bigger price for failure. It has paid the consulting fee, used precious organization time and energy, and has little to show for these expenditures when things go wrong at the end of the engagement. The disappointed organization is likely to criticize the consultant to peers and may be reluctant to undertake future consulting assignments, even when critically necessary. In extreme cases, the organization may even hold up paying fees or attempt to sue the consulting firm.

Consultants may be dissatisfied at the end of an engagement as well. Sometimes client organizations are unwilling to implement recommendations, negating the value of the engagement. The organization may not provide a good reference to prospective clients. When consultants do their best work, having a positive reference from the client is exceptionally valuable. When engagement-end problems preclude receiving future references, consultants are justifiably upset. Although rare, some consultants have taken the unusual step of suing their client at the end of an especially problematic engagement.

CONCLUSION

Hard feelings or lawsuits are no way to end any consulting engagement. The best way to avoid this unfortunate situation is to prevent it from happening by following some basic suggestions.

First, hire consultants only when internal resources are not available and be very specific about the timeframe and what is to be accomplished. Select the very best consultants, introduce them positively to the organization, and treat them with respect during the engagement. Next, keep to the mutually agreed-on timetable, communicate regularly throughout the engagement, and avoid the pitfalls that can derail any engagement. Finally, work collaboratively to end the engagement on a positive note and implement recommendations in a timely manner.

Following these suggestions will improve the probability that both organization and consultants will achieve their mutual goal of positive results from the consulting engagement.

CHAPTER FIVE

Taking Action:
The Secret of Success

THE MOST SHAMEFUL waste of healthcare dollars is money squandered on consulting reports and recommendations that are never acted on by clients. To receive the benefit from any consultation, there must be action. No matter how well-intentioned the organization or how excellent the consultant, there can be no benefit without action.

The ultimate benefit of a successful consulting engagement is positive change. An organization that improves itself is the ultimate value statement for every consultation. Two distinct components are necessary to achieve positive change. First is articulating the concept for change and improvement that is ideally suggested by consulting advice given to a receptive client. Second, and more importantly, the organization must implement the concept for change successfully. Both components for change must be present for a successful outcome to be achieved.

A consultant would not be needed if organization leaders had all the answers and knew what to do about every problem or opportunity. On the other hand, the simple presence of a capable consultant and receptive organization does not lead to successful change. Successful change comes from collaboration, with consultants contributing expertise and ideas and clients making the changes necessary to achieve a desired positive outcome. Consultants can help organizations overcome obstacles to change and find motivating factors to implement changes when change is difficult.

The best consultants do not dictate solutions to their clients or prescribe rigid formulas for change. Instead, they collaborate in such a way that the organizations themselves find the ideal solutions to problems or realize opportunities. Successful consultants understand that to be truly effective, they must help the clients help themselves. By providing a framework and processing ideas, the consultant can draw out the very best from organization leaders and encourage them to implement those ideas. In doing so, a consultant can truly help an organization grow and improve.

To illustrate, a physician with an overweight, sedentary, middle-aged patient has an opportunity to be a consultant. He can inform the patient of the risks of his lifestyle and provide ideas for improvement that make perfect sense. However, by merely informing the patient of risk factors and the consequences of failure to change, the physician is not acting as a successful consultant. If he can understand his patient well enough to motivate him to actually make lifestyle changes, for example, reminding him of his grandchildren, then he is truly acting as a consultant. If this doctor/patient collaboration actually results in changed patient behavior, then the physician has been a successful consultant.

In consulting, like medicine, knowing what to do is only part of the answer. Motivating the client to make and sustain changes completes the answer. It is this actual implementation of change that is the more difficult part. The goal of this chapter is to highlight the initiatives that lead to successful implementation.

THE IMPERATIVE OF IMPLEMENTATION

Organizations retain consultants to make positive changes. Sometimes the changes solve problems and at other times changes take advantage of an opportunity. In either case, the operative word is *change*. Organization leaders usually have a clear idea of what should be accomplished at the beginning of a consulting engagement. During the engagement, factors may arise that make things less clear and distract focus. By the end of the engagement, both consultants and organization leaders should fully envision necessary changes and a plan to successfully implement those changes.

Organizations must make a significant investment in the process leading to implementation of change. They must invest time in the consulting

process to generate ideas and concepts necessary for change. The\
money, often tens or hundreds of thousands of dollars in profes\
fees, to gain insights and expertise from consultants. And organizat\
invest considerable energy during the course of a consulting enga\
ment. Implementation is the vehicle to achieve a return for the consu\
ing investments of time and money.

Implementation value comes in many forms. A successful productivity system can save a healthcare enterprise millions of dollars, which can be reinvested to make improvements in other areas of the organization. A successfully designed new service offering can bring in new business while adding to the quality of the experience for individuals receiving care and services. A redesigned governance structure can improve the overall leadership performance of the organization. But these positive outcomes can only be achieved through change, and change is difficult under even the best of circumstances.

Positive improvements usually require change in leadership, staff, equipment, facilities, or systems. Improving productivity demands strong leaders and a highly motivated staff. Building a new outpatient surgery suite requires the investment of money and the resources to make the new facility function better than the one it replaces. Improving governance entails appointing new leaders or educating current leaders so they can perform their jobs better. No matter how brilliant a concept or improvement plan, success depends on implementing change. While consultants can help motivate organizations to change, in the final analysis, the organization itself must find the strength and purpose to implement change.

Pathway to Success: A hospital sought the expertise of a highly experienced physician consultant to help rethink the care of hip replacement patients. Hospital management staff and orthopedic surgeons had noticed wide variation in treatment plans for these patients, with some patients experiencing short lengths of stay and others experiencing extended lengths of stay. Since most of the patients were Medicare patients, the diagnostic related group (DRG) payment methodology eventually penalized the hospital for long lengths of stay.

A task force—comprising the hospital's orthopedic surgeons, nurses, operating room staff, and rehabilitation staff with the consultant as facilitator—studied "best practices" for presurgical treatment, surgical hip replacement, post-surgery care, and rehabilitation. The team quickly determined that a best practice composite could be created. They developed a hip replacement clinical pathway and published their results for all staff, nurses, and physicians involved in the care of hip replacement patients. After some fine-tuning, the pathway was implemented.

The results were dramatic. Length of stay was reduced an average of three full days, allowing patients to begin their post-surgery rehabilitation sooner and with better results, and the hospital saved over $200,000 per year. The orthopedic surgeons, many of whom made changes in their care of these patients, became convinced that patients were receiving more cost-effective and, more importantly, better care. The hospital applied the lessons learned with hip replacement patients to other types of patients. Staff was able to improve quality while reducing costs in all instances.

LEARNING FROM THE CONSULTING EXPERIENCE

In effect, the collective success of the hip replacement task force created a new approach for the hospital. The task force approach, introduced by the consultant, was used successfully to make other clinical pathway changes. The hospital received optimum value for its consulting investment by bringing people together in a nonthreatening environment to improve clinical quality, learning a new process and applying that new process to improve stroke care, knee replacements, care of congestive heart failure patients, and other clinical services.

Both an organization and its consultants should learn during each consulting engagement. A consultant is the cumulative sum of his or her experiences. Each consulting engagement, whether positive or negative, adds to the knowledge base. Organizations refine ideas, experiment with variations, and ultimately find ways to make ideas and concepts work in a new way for them. Consultants can observe and participate in this evolutionary process, which is not unlike the process of building an airplane. When a new airplane is introduced, it is the result of the cumulative knowledge of its designers. However, when the company places the plane into service, its customers identify both problems and refinements to incorporate into future models of the aircraft. Consultants, too, get feedback from their clients and change and refine their knowledge base to improve the advice and opportunities given to future clients.

Consultants bring three kinds of knowledge to their clients: technical, process, and implementation. Consultants are hired for the technical knowledge they possess to make improvements in an organization. Consultants also bring process knowledge to teach organization leaders new ways to collaborate with staff and in-house experts. If an organization learns the process, it can be applied to other areas. Ideally, consultants help organizations overcome barriers to change with their implementation knowledge. For example, if a physician resists making a change in surgical technique, an expert consultant can often overcome that resistance by citing a dozen examples, from personal experience, in which surgeons have made similar changes with successful results. Resistance to change works best in a vacuum. Consultants can fill the vacuum with experience and give even those most resistant to change the knowledge they need to consider alternatives.

ENSURING VALUE

Successful consultants add value to the organizations they serve by imparting these three types of knowledge and by enabling organizations to use the knowledge to successfully implement change. Although good consultants possess technical, process, and implementation knowledge, it is how they interact and collaborate with their clients that determines whether value is provided to the clients. If knowledge were the sole determining factor of leadership success, Jimmy Carter would have been one of the greatest U.S. presidents. That he was not is an example of the inability of technical knowledge, in and of itself, to inspire great achievements. Consultants, too, can have real knowledge and still fail as consultants. Successful consultants have the ability to transfer knowledge and then inspire clients to do great things with that knowledge.

Value is found in successful activity. A large contributor to successful action is receptiveness in both consultants and clients. Organizations can contribute technical and process insights, and consultants should be receptive to learning from them. If the consultants are open to learning from clients, they can absorb what they learn and refine it based on their own experiences. This combination can bring forth new ideas that suit their clients' needs best. Organizations eager, or at least willing, to learn from their consultants will benefit from their openness. Organizations can also absorb the technical and process expertise of their consultants and refine it for their own use. Clients and consultants collaborating together create the most important knowledge component of all—implementation knowledge—when making positive changes in organizations.

Ensuring value can also be viewed in an economic context if the value of services received from the consultant was worth the investment in consulting fees. As the engagement reaches an end, and implementation begins, the economic value can be both short- and long-term in nature.

> **Task Forces Revisited:** A nursing home was faced with the prospect of losing a million dollars in the coming fiscal year. Previously, the nursing home had experienced modest profits, and its management team considered itself adept at keeping costs as low as possible. Senior management evaluated several different consulting firms to assist with reducing costs. After concluding that the "slash and burn" and the "benchmark" approaches were not compatible with the organization, the nursing home chose a small consulting firm whose specialty was organizing management teams to look hard at their own costs and challenging them to make changes without relying on outside benchmark databases or superficial cookie-cutter solutions.
>
> The consultant's simple approach was to organize the management team into multidisciplinary task forces. In the past, the nursing home had formed task forces along organization lines, teaming nursing leaders, technical department leaders, and so forth. The consultant made sure that task forces were organized so that nursing, technical, and support department leaders served on the same task force. Then these multidisciplinary task forces were asked to challenge each other to arrive at the cost-reduction goal.
>
> The nursing home's management team experienced a revelation during this process. They got to know each other better and they challenged each other successfully. Brainstorming sessions produced creative ideas that ultimately saved one million dollars when implemented, more than enough to restore profitability. But more important than the financial success was the success of the multidisciplinary task force approach. It was so successful that the nursing home was able to forego the use of a "customer service" consultant the following year. Instead, the nursing home reorganized the multidisciplinary task forces and used the same approach to successfully identify ways to improve customer service

throughout the facility. This organization received excellent value for the cost-reduction engagement, and it received ongoing value by reusing the multidisciplinary task forces to avoid subsequent consulting expenses.

POST-CONSULTATION ALTERNATIVES

Organizations and consultants should both be interested in whether an engagement achieves desired outcomes. However, when a consulting engagement ends, it is not always clear whether the desired outcome will be achieved. The organization must implement recommended changes to achieve desired results after the consultants have completed their work. It is not uncommon for weeks, months, or even years to pass before it can be clearly established whether an engagement was successful.

Organization leaders can determine if the terms of the engagement have been fulfilled at the end of the consultation. Both the organization and its consultants should continually monitor their respective commitments for completion. Although the consultants have an obligation to provide their deliverables, how can both the organization and consultants determine if the engagement was ultimately successful in implementation?

The best way to truly measure success or failure in a consulting engagement is by post-engagement follow-ups. Depending on the type of consulting and implementation timetable, follow-up visits by the consultants three and six months after the engagement ends are valuable. Bringing the consultants back to compare expected versus actual results of recommended changes is a sound approach for both clients and consultants. Organization leaders will determine if the consultants' recommendations worked as planned. The consultants will discern whether the clients implemented the recommendations properly to achieve full benefits. Unexpected issues and challenges—or even benefits—can arise during implementation.

When consultants work with an organization post-implementation to determine the level of success, they often add further insights that may be beneficial for the organization. Just as often, consultants gain valuable insights useful for advising future clients. Both consultants and organizations must be aware of the tendency of organizations to regress after changes are implemented. No engagement can be considered successful if needed changes are achieved only on a short-term basis. The ability of an organization to sustain successful change is a function of management's commitment and capability. If management falls short, there can be no real value imparted to the organization.

> **Staff Reduction Fiasco:** An urban hospital's leaders knew it was substantially overstaffed. They hired a consulting firm with expertise in productivity management and fringe benefit programs for employees to assist with creating a staff reduction approach that would not violate its "no layoffs" commitment to employees.
>
> After thorough analysis of staffing patterns, it was determined that over 100 employees needed to go. The consultants designed an early retirement offer to encourage employees to leave voluntarily. The program was very successful, and nearly 150 employees took the early retirement option. Unfortunately, they were not in the departments that the hospital and consultants knew were overstaffed. The early retirement program cost the hospital several million dollars to implement.
>
> One year later, the hospital's overall staffing was back at the level where it had been before the early retirement offer. The consultants blamed the chief executive for poor implementation. The chief executive blamed the consultants for giving poor advice. This was truly a fiasco for the organization. It nearly went bankrupt before it got control of the situation and implemented the layoffs it had so strenuously tried to avoid.

PROVIDING CONSTRUCTIVE FEEDBACK TO CONSULTANTS

It is in everyone's best interest to hold a constructive feedback session at the end of a consulting engagement. Consultants can use constructive feedback to improve their services to future clients. The organization benefits from the process because it encourages the organization to assess its own performance during the engagement.

At the end of the engagement, consultants should perform an exit interview with all of the organization's staff that worked with them. This interview should provide the consultants with the client's viewpoints on their strengths, weaknesses, and areas where the client believes the consultants could improve. Consultants should encourage their clients to provide critical feedback with the benefit of hindsight. Answering the question, "If we were starting the engagement all over again today, what could we do better?" is especially insightful. Excellent consultants will take great pains to encourage their clients to provide insights, especially on how things might be improved in future engagements.

Consultants, too, should provide clients with their insights at the end of the engagement. Consultants are in an excellent position to offer feedback on the organization's strengths, weaknesses, and areas for improvement. An organization that truly wishes to improve itself will actively seek the consultants' feedback on how to perform more effectively. The value of this feedback is enhanced if both client and consultants are completely candid with each other. This presumes that by the end of a successful engagement, sufficient mutual trust and respect exist for candor to be encouraged.

Organization leaders must also be willing to have a candid discussion with the consultants about the financial value of the engagement. "Was it worth the fee?" is the question excellent consultants want to know but may be afraid to ask. The full value of a successful engagement may not be apparent until some time after the engagement is over, which also encourages a post-engagement follow-up meeting three to six months after the engagement is concluded. The organization will more likely determine the full and fair value of the engagement in the interim based on the success or failure of implementing the consultants' recommendations. Clients and consultants should work hard to ensure that the end of the engagement is a positive experience for both parties.

CREATING A POSITIVE "LAST IMPRESSION"

It is principally the consultants' obligation to ensure that they make a positive "last impression" on their clients and that the engagement ends on a positive note. The consultants should ascertain if all of their engagement commitments and contractual obligations are accomplished. Consultants should, whenever possible, seek to add additional value to the engagement by providing "extras" not required in the consulting agreement where feasible. These extras might take the form of providing additional meetings at no expense to the client or performing additional services at no charge. Consultants should always send courtesy thank you letters to those individuals with whom they worked closely during the engagement.

Organizations, too, should work at ensuring that a positive last impression is achieved with the consultants. Public acknowledgement of the consultants' contributions during key meetings is always appreciated. Post-engagement thank you letters are rarely sent but also much appreciated by consultants. Paying final bills on time creates a positive impression. Most importantly, willingness to serve as a future reference for the consultants is perhaps the greatest compliment of all.

Excellent consultants often become attached to their clients. Consultants often feel slightly let down when an engagement is over, especially if it has been long and challenging. A public thank you or private expression of appreciation is never sought, but always fondly remembered by consultants. Positive last impressions can go a long way toward establishing long-lasting professional and even personal relationships between consultants and clients.

CONCLUSION

No consulting report ever accomplished anything of value by itself. Value is achieved when organizations do something positive with the consultants' recommendations. Success is measured not by the elegance of the report but by the success the client achieves after being inspired by and following the report's recommendations.

Consultants are like physicians—they can be generalists or specialists. No one consultant, or consulting firm for that matter, could hope to accumulate enough knowledge to successfully advise all healthcare enterprises on all matters. Logical groupings of consultants and their services exist, just as do specialty physicians.

Part Two, "Consultants for Governing Boards," explores in detail the kinds of consultants available to healthcare boards and how to get the best work and value from their services.

PART TWO

*Consultants for
Governing Boards*

CHAPTER SIX

Board Performance Improvement

S UCCESS AND FAILURE of a healthcare enterprise begin in the boardroom. Although the constructive use of consultants to improve governance performance is in its infancy, this is an area of great opportunity for those organizations that wish to truly improve governance performance.

If healthcare chief executives perform poorly, they are fired. If clinicians or non-clinical staff are incompetent, they too are asked to leave. But healthcare boards can perform so poorly that their organizations are forced into bankruptcy, yet the boards are rarely, if ever, held accountable. Because of this lack of accountability, boards rarely focus on their own performance—and their organizations can pay a high price for this neglect. The revelations surrounding the failure of governance at the Enron Corporation, for example, illustrate clearly how inattentive or ineffective boards can wreak havoc on even the largest organizations.

Governing board performance is by far the most neglected performance aspect of nearly all healthcare organizations. Why is this the case? Many reasons exist, but ego and misinterpreted reality are high on the list. Healthcare boards are populated with highly intelligent people, but many are not properly trained to apply leadership skills in this unique governance position. They may inadvertently set aside business and life experiences that would serve them well in the boardroom.

Healthcare boards often spend tens of thousands of dollars on financial audits, hundreds of thousands of dollars per year on legal services, and, in some circumstances, millions of dollars on turnaround consultants. However, when it comes to evaluating and improving their own performance, many governing boards grudgingly devote only a few thousand dollars for an annual weekend board retreat and feel satisfied they received sufficient education to perform their governance role satisfactorily.

Nothing could be further from the truth. Countless healthcare organizations have failed because of poorly performing governing boards. Although excuses such as competition, regulations, and patient/payer mix are often given for the failure, inadequate boards are more likely the cause. Bankruptcy, merger, and sale have all been used as exit strategies by failing healthcare governing boards. Government regulations, managed care, or competition may be blamed for an organization's failure, yet boards are rarely held responsible.

The governing board sets the overall performance standard for a healthcare organization. If good members are selected and trained well, governance duties are performed well. Good governance consistently seeks ways to improve the organization, and achieves success no matter how onerous the government regulations, how poor the reimbursement, or how many competitors occupy the organization's marketplace. Governing boards need to spend more time and more money evaluating their own performance and taking appropriate actions to improve that performance. They must have the courage to admit shortcomings and the conviction to address governance problems. No matter how big the egos in the boardroom, every board member must seek to improve his or her personal performance in addition to the board's overall performance. The board must be as accountable as the hospital's chief executive and senior management. Just because the board is made up of volunteers is not an excuse for poor performance.

WHEN TO RETAIN A GOVERNANCE CONSULTANT

No matter its size, ownership structure, or location, every healthcare organization should have a governance performance "check up" using an independent consultant. The frequency of such a consultation could be debated, but not the absolute necessity. At a minimum, this performance audit should take place every five years. Every three years would be more effective.

Governing boards would never consider foregoing the organization's annual financial audit. Why, then, do most boards fail to audit their own performance? Perhaps it is a fear of criticism. Maybe they are insecure in their role, or simply ignorant about the necessity to periodically audit governance performance. Whatever the reason, one of the greatest opportunities for improving the performance of healthcare organizations begins with the governing board.

Double Dipping: A large community hospital retained an experienced governance consultant to evaluate the performance of the chief executive officer and the governing board. Both parties felt that the performance of the other could be considerably improved. After conducting interviews with board members and senior management, it became evident to the consultant that both parties were right. Performance was lacking and there was considerable room for improvement on both sides.

The central problem for both board and chief executive was conflict of interest. Several members of the board were obviously using their board membership for personal gain. One owned a construction company and received millions of dollars in contracts from the hospital without competitive bidding. Another ran the telephone service that the hospital purchased, again without any competitive bidding. Still another was the head of the law firm that handled all of the hospital's legal business.

Management also had problems. The chief executive was paid a well-below-market salary. Board members seemed to be very proud of this fact. The chief executive did not seem to mind the low salary either. This puzzled the consultant until he discovered that the chief executive had coerced most senior management and half of the department heads to work as his personal sales force in a household products marketing company. All were using hospital time to sell products to hospital employees. The chief executive received a percentage of all sales, more than compensating for his below-market salary.

When the consultant pointed out that both the board and chief executive would have to discontinue these unethical practices, the board chair fired the consultant. The consultant concluded that some boards and chief executives deserve each other.

Aside from periodically auditing governing board performance, governing boards have many other opportunities to use independent consultants. If chief executive officer turnover is high, poor governing board performance may be a contributing factor. Instead of recruiting a new chief executive every two or three years, it would be better to retain a governance consultant to explore the root issues. Another opportune time to take a critical look at the governing board is during a prolonged period of poor financial performance. In addition to approving management's recommendation for a cost-reduction consulting engagement, the governing board should consider spending a portion of that amount assessing its own performance. Independent governance consultants can help with any number of specific challenges such as managing board officer succession, resolving conflicts of interest, and structuring committees for maximum effectiveness.

Consultants may also be used for recruiting new board members. While board recruitment has long been an informal process, conducting a professional search for board members is gaining popularity. Education and development is another area where independent consultants can be useful to governing boards. A weekend board retreat, however, is not sufficient education. To be effective, education and development require continuous investment of board time throughout the year.

Another clear opportunity for governance consulting is when the organization faces a turnaround situation. Turnarounds are not only failures of management, but also of the board. Boards should bear a large share of the responsibility when an organization becomes so distressed that a turnaround is necessary. The start of an effective turnaround should begin with changing the healthcare organization's board leadership. Firing management without making necessary board-level changes will not automatically make the turnaround successful in the long term.

Consultation to healthcare governing boards is severely underused. Boards should spend at least as much time and money on their own performance improvement as they do on their organization's annual financial audit. Board members must make a commitment to apply the same high standards to themselves as they apply to the rest of the organization. Opportunity for improvement is almost limitless. Committing to excellence can transform terrible boards into adequate boards, adequate boards into exemplary boards, and exemplary boards into role models for organizational leadership. No greater opportunity exists for reward in healthcare than using high quality consultation to improve the performance of governing boards.

DEFINING THE SCOPE OF ENGAGEMENT

How does the board start once it realizes the necessity for improving governance performance? Before defining the scope of an engagement for a governance performance consultant, a governing board must decide who will retain the consultant. This is the first test of a board's commitment to improve its own performance, since unanimity in the decision to retain a consultant is unlikely. Several options exist. Officers on the executive committee and other key leaders may be given the authority to retain a governance consultant. The board chair could retain the consultant, ideally with the concurrence of a majority of board members. Perhaps most controversially, the chief executive officer may be given the authority to retain a governance consultant with, or without, the concurrence of the majority of the board. After all, the chief executive officer is often in the best position to identify when a governance performance consultant is necessary.

The next step in retaining a governance performance consultant is to define the scope of the consulting engagement. The five elements in the scope of any governance performance improvement consultation include:

1. assessing current weaknesses;
2. identifying performance improvement sources;
3. deliberating alternatives;
4. gaining consensus on desired improvements; and
5. developing an implementation action plan.

Include all five elements in a governance performance improvement consultation, particularly emphasizing deliberation of alternatives and consensus around desired improvements. A sample engagement scope of a governance performance improvement follows.

Assessing Current Weaknesses

The governing board desires to evaluate its performance in all areas of governance and to implement strategies to improve its performance and set a positive example for the organization as a whole. At a minimum, the following aspects shall be carefully evaluated:

- Board organization and committees
- Trustee selection and orientation
- Trustee job description and performance expectations
- Conflict of interest expectations
- Continuing education and officer succession planning
- Confidentiality requirements
- Governance policies

Identifying Performance Improvement Sources

The consultant will review governance policies, minutes of governing board and committee meetings for the previous 12 months, and all internal and external reports relevant to the performance of the board (e.g., JCAHO accreditation reports, financial audit, strategic plan). The consultant will attend, as guest observer, two board meetings and four committee meetings to gain firsthand knowledge of the board in action. In addition, the consultant will interview all board members, senior management, and medical staff leaders to gain their insights.

Deliberating Alternatives

Based on the review of background material, attendance at key meetings, and personal interviews, the consultant will assess the board's strengths and weaknesses, provide several initial ideas for performance improvement, and develop preliminary recommendations that will be presented to the board for further refinement and discussion.

Gaining Consensus on Desired Improvements

The consultant will facilitate further discussion among the board members to build consensus on the desired initiatives for governance performance improvement. Although unanimity may not be achievable, consensus is absolutely critical.

Developing an Implementation Action Plan

In conjunction with the chief executive and board leaders, the consultant will prepare an action plan that identifies specific initiatives, a defined timeframe, and follow-up actions to implement the desired governance performance improvements.

A full request for proposal sample (RFP), using this scope of engagement, is provided in Appendix C. The RFP sample can be adapted to practically any type of governance consultation by changing the scope of engagement section.

Once an RFP has been prepared, the board's attention shifts to selecting the best governance consultant to meet its performance improvement needs.

SELECTING THE BEST GOVERNANCE CONSULTANT

Various governance consultant options exist. Many large accounting and consulting firms dedicate divisions or individuals to advising boards. A number of small specialty firms and solo practitioners focus on healthcare governing boards as well. Although some healthcare chief executives who were fired or otherwise unsuccessful have promoted themselves as governing board consultants, they are not usually good candidates for providing advice on how to improve governance.

A well-crafted RFP is essential to select a good governance consultant. The importance of thorough reference checking, even more so than for other types of consultation, cannot be overemphasized. Several desired characteristics of governance consultants should be considered when evaluating alternatives. The most important characteristic of a governance advisor is absolute honesty. Boards that have performance problems need objective advice, even if the advice hurts some feelings. Most boards have talented and successful members who may have egos to match their successes. A consultant who is in the least intimidated by members of a board will not serve his or her client successfully. It is not easy to find a consultant with this characteristic, but it is well worth the search.

A second desired characteristic is personal governance experience and a track record of motivating boards to change ineffective practices. Most governance consultants can give an entertaining weekend retreat. It takes greater skill to work with a board over time to change its errant ways.

Being a good listener is still another trait of an effective governance consultant. Perhaps that is why some former chief executive officers fail when they set out to be governance consultants. They are more skilled in talking than in listening.

Creativity and the ability to elicit creativity in others are also desired characteristics of a good governance consultant. The abilities to develop alternatives for debate and discussion and adapt ideas from other governance settings are part of this trait. The ability to help a board reach consensus is another desired characteristic. With consensus building comes the knowledge that it may not be possible or even desirable to achieve complete unanimity for a particular course of action.

Independence is another important characteristic in an excellent governance consultant. A board should not have to worry that its consultant is not being candid because the consultant feels future consulting work might be lost by being honest. For that reason, it is advisable to disqualify any consulting firms currently retained for accounting or management issues from providing governance performance advice.

Each of these characteristics should be kept in mind when healthcare boards evaluate RFP responses for governance improvement consultation. At least three consultants should receive the RFP and at least two of the respondents should be selected for personal interviews by board leaders. Reference checks are important to identify the consultants selected for personal interviews. Personal interviews with several excellent finalists selected for consideration should give board leaders the ability to select the consultant most capable of performing the consultation and working effectively with the board to implement positive changes in governance performance. Once the selection decision has been made, the next step is to prepare the board for a successful experience.

LAYING THE GROUNDWORK FOR A SUCCESSFUL OUTCOME

As simple as it sounds, motivation to improve is key to a successful governance performance improvement consultation. Strong motivation in a few board leaders will set the stage for the rest of the board to seek positive change. The board must also be open and honest in their communication with the consultant. By being completely candid, with themselves and the consultant, board members will enhance their ability to identify governance strengths and shortcomings.

A strong commitment of time is another factor for success. The consultant must have sufficient time to study the board and elicit its successes and challenges. Even more importantly, enough time must be set aside during the consulting engagement for meaningful discussion and consideration of alternatives. Governance improvement opportunities are often hidden. They do, however, emerge during thoughtful discussion and debates as the merits of various improvement initiatives are fully explored and refined.

Perhaps the most difficult factor for success in governance improvement is the ability to face shortcomings and to make necessary changes. It is not enough to know what to do—the board must have the fortitude to do it. Although the consultant can help the board develop a good plan for performance improvement, only the board itself can implement the plan. Commitment to implementing the plan is the final determining factor of a successful governance engagement.

> **Improvement by Policy:** A large urban hospital experienced an up-and-down record of financial performance over a ten-year period. Some years were profitable; other years had operating losses. Toward the end of the 10-year roller-coaster ride, the hospital entered a period when its losses mounted to such an extent it faced possible closure. The board retained an independent consultant to evaluate governance, believing that the failure of the organization to succeed was in large measure due to the board's own performance. This kind of insight is extraordinarily rare in healthcare boards.
>
> The board members' intuition was correct. They had indeed done a poor job governing the organization. During declining periods of performance, they accepted management's superficial excuses for financial problems. They did not critically evaluate the chief executive. They let medical staff leaders abdicate their responsibility for quality oversight. The end result was an organization with poor leadership, poor financial performance, and poor medical quality. For some organizations, this would be the end of the story.
>
> The governance performance consultant helped board members begin a complete governance overhaul. They reorganized the board by replacing officers, updating the committee structure, and completely

revamping the reporting and accountability systems for management. Then, they went one step further: they solidified their governance overhaul by writing a comprehensive set of governance policies, spelling out in great detail the duties and responsibilities of the board.

This governing board had the courage and conviction to face its worst performance problems and fix them. Board members were subsequently rewarded for their foresight. Instead of closing the hospital, the board went on to oversee the revitalization of management and the medical staff. The organization survived, due in no small measure to the ability of the board to improve its own performance. With comprehensive policies and standards in place, the hospital will never again face the prospect of bankruptcy and closure due to governance shortcomings.

GOVERNANCE POLICIES

Various regulatory agencies require healthcare governing boards to periodically review and approve formal organization plans. Healthcare organizations develop emergency management plans, biohazard plans, compliance plans, quality improvement plans, and so forth. The list is nearly endless, but it rarely includes a governance plan.

The end result of a governance performance evaluation should be the creation of a comprehensive governance plan. The plan should include a board mission statement, compatible with the organization's mission statement, and a governance policy manual that outlines the board's structure and organization. At a minimum, a governance policy manual should include:

- governance policies;
- communication policies;
- chief executive policies;
- finance and planning policies; and
- quality of care policies.

These policies should set forth the responsibilities and expectations of the board and the chief executive. The policy manual gives the board a benchmark against which it can measure its performance. A sample table of contents for a comprehensive governance policy manual and several sample governance policies are provided in Appendix D.

RETREATING FROM RETREATS

Governance by retreat is a common pitfall that should be avoided by boards. Although retreats can be fun and even mildly productive, a board cannot improve itself by merely having a weekend educational retreat. Typically, board retreats are held in nice surroundings with an outside speaker slotted in between golf and cocktails. Some retreat speakers are extraordinarily entertaining, and it is not uncommon for retreat speakers to whip board members into a frenzy of positive emotions and high expectations. On Monday morning, however, the consultant flies to the next retreat and the board will likely revert to its previous behavior.

Some progressive organizations have abandoned the annual weekend board retreat with outside speakers in favor of "in-house" retreats featuring their own experts. Vice presidents, chiefs of medical departments, departmental directors, and nursing leaders represent a wealth of healthcare expertise. A typical agenda might include the chief of radiology discussing coming improvements in imaging technology; the chief of obstetrics presenting a plan for improving quality; the vice president of patient care discussing the challenges of retaining qualified nurses; and the rehabilitation department director reviewing planned programs for treating injured workers more effectively.

Healthcare boards should consider in-house expert retreats as a cheaper and more educational alternative to consultant retreats. The money saved could be invested in a governance performance evaluation, a much more effective use of consulting dollars.

PITFALLS TO AVOID IN GOVERNANCE CONSULTATION

A common pitfall in governance performance consulting is expecting too much too soon. Boards that desire to truly improve their performance must be prepared to spend the time and money to achieve improvements. Governance consultants are not miracle workers. They cannot transform a poorly functioning board into an effective one over the weekend or even over a few months.

Another pitfall is expecting the consultant to fire a poorly performing chief executive or ask a problematic board member to step down. The board is responsible for hiring, firing, and retiring, not its consultants.

Crossover consulting is another problem that can surface when a large accounting or management consulting firm provides governance consulting. It is extremely difficult for governance consultants to act truly independent if their firm performs the yearly financial audit or other lucrative management consulting services for the organization.

A subtle pitfall to avoid is the lack of complete honesty, either on the part of the organization or the consultant. For example, it is difficult for a consultant to tell the board chairman, who is also the president of the local bank, that he is an ineffective leader, even if it is painfully obvious. However, it must be done for the good of the organization. It is just as difficult for a chief executive to share a discovery that an important board member totally ignores the conflict of interest policy. For a successful consultation to take place, complete candor must be the rule of the day.

One of the most critical pitfalls is never getting started on a governance improvement consultation. A myriad of excuses are often heard: "We can't spend the money ... We're already doing a great job ... Board members will never change their ways ... We'll never agree." These excuses are extremely compelling, and it is still rare that a board retains a good consultant to truly assess its performance and recommend improvements. Board performance is just as important as a healthcare organization's financial or clinical performance. Time and money must be spent to periodically get an unbiased professional opinion on how to improve it. The outcome of the effort will be better-organized governing boards that are much better prepared to discharge their duties.

CHECKLIST FOR SUCCESSFUL GOVERNANCE PERFORMANCE IMPROVEMENT

Governance improvement is not complicated. For boards to improve, they must first objectively evaluate their performance. Every healthcare governing board benefits from thoroughly and thoughtfully reviewing its own performance and implementing improvements in its governance process.

Every governing board also benefits from regular education. Boards should invest more time and money on themselves than they have in the past, elevating the importance of improving governance quality to the level of importance of quality care and fiscal responsibility in the organization. A checklist for a successful governance performance consultation includes the following actions.

1. *Evaluate.* Commit time and money to hire a governance consultant at least every five years to independently evaluate board performance.
2. *Be honest.* Be honest in seeking and listening to meaningful critiques of board performance and suggestions for improvement.
3. *Implement.* Implement improvements at the conclusion of the performance evaluation.
4. *Take responsibility.* Take full responsibility for setting the leadership tone for the organization.
5. *Articulate.* Create a comprehensive governance plan and policy manual articulating expectations and performance improvement goals.
6. *Commit.* Continually improve performance through a commitment to education and periodic evaluations to ensure the board is not straying from performance standards.

CONCLUSION

Governance performance improvement should be a priority for all health-care boards. The constructive use of consultants can be very helpful in the education, evaluation, and performance improvement of boards. When boards function at an optimal level of performance, they can make well-informed decisions, including those concerning consultants. As the Enron debacle has demonstrated, ineffective governing boards can be the downfall of any organization, and failure to oversee outside consultants, such as auditors, can be a significant factor in their demise.

CHAPTER SEVEN

Certified Public Accountants

ALMOST EVERY HEALTHCARE organization uses the services of a certified public accountant to annually audit financial statement efficacy. Unfortunately, many boards do not periodically evaluate the quality of their outside auditors. Also, unfortunately, some boards do not really understand how to get the "full story" from their accountants and rely instead on template reports and superficial presentations. This chapter focuses on annual financial audit services prepared for the healthcare organization's governing board. It will explain the choices available, how to select the best auditor, and how to evaluate and get the most value from audit services.

Many healthcare governing boards have abdicated fiduciary responsibility by adopting a passive attitude toward annual financial audits. These boards may retain auditors who are not really independent because of overlapping consulting relationships, ask few or no questions when things go wrong, and look for external excuses when their organizations decline. Certified public accountants performing the audit function are one of the most important types of consultants retained by healthcare governing boards. Unfortunately, boards commonly delegate their selection to senior management. While senior management should be involved in the selection process, they should not control it. Financial consulting services delivered to management are covered in Chapter 12.

Board members need to know what the limitations of their auditors are and how to ask focused questions to receive full value from their outside auditor's services. A well-informed board, asking thoughtful questions and working with a thorough and honest auditor, is the best possible combination. Unfortunately, this combination rarely occurs in healthcare organizations. It is far more common for board members of a failing organization to ask what went wrong after the fact. They attempt to blame their auditors and demand to know why there was no warning of impending doom. Boards may even go to the extreme of suing the auditors, as if that would restore life to a bankrupt organization. On the other hand, it is just as common for auditors to be reluctant to share concerns they may have about financial statements or the financial staff of the organization they are auditing. Many auditors follow a "don't ask, don't tell" motto.

In today's environment of ever-increasing mergers and consolidations among accounting firms, the line between financial audit services and consulting services is becoming blurred at best. This has given rise to conflicts of interest within some of the large accounting firms. The very real dilemma these firms face is how to be forthright on audit reports to an organization while avoiding the risk that honesty might anger management enough to disqualify the firm from lucrative consulting projects in the future.

As with any consulting service, for a healthcare organization to receive quality and value from their investment in consulting dollars, the organization needs to be well-informed, ask excellent questions, and seek honesty and integrity from the accounting firm responsible for its annual audit. To accept less is to open the door to superficial auditing service, which can contribute to the failure of the organization. Several high-profile healthcare organization bankruptcies in the 1990s confirmed this sad fact. More recently, the audit firm involvement in the largest corporate bankruptcy in U.S. history points out the dangers that occur when the integrity of the outside auditors is compromised. The objective of this chapter is to define what is needed from the audit firm and to offer practical advice to governing boards to avoid the many pitfalls that plague this consultant/client relationship.

CHOICES FOR ACCOUNTING SERVICES

Fortunately for healthcare organizations, there are many excellent choices available for accounting audit services. The "big" accounting firms are the most well-known. In past years it was the "big eight." Then it became the "big six." Currently it is the "big five." Mergers and consolidations have shrunk the number of "bigs," but they still are the dominant providers of audit services to the healthcare industry.

The big accounting firms offer healthcare clients great depth of professional staff and national expertise. They have the necessary resources to provide services to even the largest healthcare organizations. They offer diversified services, including many types of consulting services, in addition to traditional accounting and audit services. They have offices throughout the United States, serving large urban medical centers, small rural hospitals, and every conceivable size of healthcare organization in between.

Another choice for accounting and audit services is a specialty accounting firm focused on the healthcare industry. These firms tend to be regional in nature and offer many of the same services as the "bigs" without the national scope of practice. Regional specialty firms usually offer a wide variety of consulting services in addition to traditional accounting and audit services. They typically have multiple offices in a geographic region and can call on the resources of their individual offices for the benefit of healthcare clients, much the same as the "bigs" do.

A third option, used most often in smaller communities, is the local accounting firm. While a local firm does not have all of the resources of a "big" or regional firm, some healthcare organizations believe the personalized service of a local firm outweighs the absence of regional or national healthcare expertise.

All of these choices for audit services have one major drawback: potential conflicts of interest. For the "big" and specialty firms, providing other kinds of consulting services can be very problematic from an ethical standpoint. For example, candor in an audit report can be compromised if the accounting firm is selling a consulting engagement worth three times the audit engagement in professional fees. This dilemma occurs frequently because of the mergers and consolidations in accounting firms. Conflicts of interest can be present with local firms, too. It is not uncommon for partners in local accounting firms to be on the governing board of their community's hospital, which again raises an integrity issue. For example, does the local firm feel compelled to soften its audit comments so as not to embarrass a partner who is on the board? Are auditors reluctant to be forthright because it may cause their firm to lose an otherwise lucrative client? You should be very conscious of these potential conflicts of interest and actively take steps to avoid them. Clearly defining the expectations for auditors is the first step.

DEFINING THE ANNUAL AUDIT

More thought should be given to defining the scope of engagement for annual audit services than is usually done. Complacency is also a problem with accounting and audit services. The same firm is commonly rehired year after year to perform the annual audit with little or no due diligence on the part of board or management. At the same time, little or no thought is given to what the annual financial audit should cover. This indifference can lead to big trouble.

The content and format of audit services provided by accounting firms are somewhat prescribed by current accounting regulations and practice. A full audit should contain the following seven components:

1. Required communications
2. Report of the independent auditor (opinion letter)
3. Balance sheet
4. Statement of operations
5. Statement of cash flows
6. Notes to the financial statements
7. Management letter

The introduction to the audit includes the required communications and opinion letter. The required communications are a series of statements required by the Generally Accepted Auditing Standards (GAAS). The opinion letter is designed to give basic assurances to the governing board that accounting systems are sound and that the financial statements accurately represent the financial health of the organization. However, because opinion letters have become filled with qualifying statements, their content has become almost meaningless. Opinion letters are offered with three major conclusions. A "clean" or "unqualified" opinion letter gives assurance to the board that financial statements accurately characterize the status of the organization. A "qualified" opinion letter specifies a particular area in which financial results are questioned. A "going concern" opinion letter expresses doubt as to whether or not the organization will still be in business one year and a day following the issuance of the letter. Obviously, organizations seek to receive unqualified opinion letters from their auditors.

The financial statement sections of the audit consist of the balance sheet, statements of operations and cash flows, and notes sections. Financial statements should accurately represent the financial health of the organization. Problems can occur in interpreting financial results, however, especially when they are poor. Accounting firms do not like to deliver bad news. They especially do not like to make chief executives or chief financial officers look bad. Often they forget that the board, not management, is the client and present financial statements in such a way as to minimize the bad news. This happens all too frequently in healthcare. Judging by shareholder suits against audit firms, it happens in the for-profit business world as well. Governing boards must take active steps to ensure that their annual audit is delivered objectively.

The management letter section of the annual audit identifies systems or people problems within the financial operations of the organization that need attention or corrective action. The quality of the management letter varies widely from superficial to thoughtful and analytical reports. The difference in quality is often the result of defining the engagement scope.

Bad News Dilemma: A large urban hospital used the audit services of one of the "big five" accounting firms. The hospital had used the firm for both audit and consulting services for seven consecutive years. During a multi-year period of declining financial performance, the hospital received unqualified audit opinion letters. The auditors raised no concerns during their brief annual meetings with the board. During the entire seven-year period no personal meetings took place between the audit firm leaders and leaders of the board.

Even while the financial position of the hospital was deteriorating significantly, the board had no private contact with the auditors. The auditors' annual presentation of audit results met with no questions from the board. After an especially bad year of financial performance, the audit firm partner requested a private, personal meeting with the board chairman to express his concerns about the chief executive and chief financial officer.

The board chairman, upon hearing the partner's concerns, defended the senior executives and refused to initiate any corrective actions with the executives. During the next year, the hospital's financial performance deteriorated to critical levels. The audit partner then met with the Catholic sponsors of the hospital to express his concerns directly. The sponsors communicated these concerns to the board chairman, who, instead of acting responsibly, became extremely angry with the audit firm and threatened to fire it. The sponsor intervened and fired the chief executive officer and forced the board chairman to resign.

In hindsight, both the governing board and Catholic sponsors of this hospital concluded that they had failed in their fiduciary responsibilities by not insisting on regular private contact with the audit firm. The hospital subsequently underwent a turnaround, barely surviving the ordeal.

EXPECTATIONS FOR AUDITORS

At a bare minimum, a governing board should expect its annual audit to meet applicable accounting standards. That bare minimum is only a foundation, however—much more should be expected.

In addition to the mandated reviews and reports, the scope of the engagement for a thorough annual audit review should include:

- communication expectations;
- mid-year follow-up review;
- periodic special analysis reports; and
- integrity expectations.

Communication expectations for the audit should specify that the auditor meet with the chief executive and chief financial officer during the review and preparation of draft reports. Other expected communications should occur between the auditor and the board chair and the chair of the board's finance committee before audit results are finalized. These should be private meetings and should provide the opportunity for board leaders to carefully query the accounting firm about the review and the financial status of the organization. Questions that should be asked in these private sessions include the following:

1. How confident are you that these financial statements accurately represent the organization's true financial status?
2. How well-prepared were the organization's accounting staff and senior management for the audit?

3. Do you have any concerns about the quality of the senior accounting staff, chief financial officer, or chief executive officer?
4. If you were a member of the governing board, what concerns would you have about finances for the coming year?
5. Are any follow-up reports or analysis statements necessary based on your assessment of our organization?

After these private interviews, the audit firm should provide draft reports and oral presentations to the finance committee and full board. Only after these meetings have taken place should the audit report be finalized. The accounting firm should take great care to invite questions from the finance committee and board members.

Mid-year follow-up reviews are another expectation that should be included in the scope of the annual financial audit. Typically, after the audit is presented to the board, no contact takes place until the next year's audit. The audit firm should be required to return six months after presenting audit results to assess the organization's progress in correcting problems identified in the audit or resolving operational problems that are causing the organization to perform poorly.

Governing boards should also look to their audit firms to periodically perform special analysis projects beyond the reports required for the actual audit. Special reports you may request of the auditors in the course of the year could include:

- accounts receivable process integrity;
- contractual allowance methodology integrity;
- fraud/theft exposure;
- purchasing policy effectiveness and consistency;
- cash management integrity; and
- physician contracting status.

An annual audit covers only the bare minimum and cannot offer the board complete comfort as to the financial status of the organization. Effective governing boards know they should be probing below the surface of their annual reports. Those areas listed above have been responsible for the demise of many healthcare organizations during the past decade and should receive a special review every three or four years.

Finally, members of the audit firm should be completely honest and candid with the board at all times. More than one organization has been undone by a failure on the part of the audit firm to be completely candid.

Tax Man Cometh: A struggling inner-city hospital underwent a five-year period of steadily declining financial performance. The organization's auditor, a "big five" accounting firm, provided accounting and consulting services throughout the period. It presented an unqualified opinion letter following its fifth audit to the board. The finance committee did not ask a single question, even though the financial statements clearly showed a loss of massive proportions for the fourth straight year.

One month following the audit, the Internal Revenue Service placed a lien on the hospital's assets due to non-payment of federal withholding payroll taxes. Chaos followed. After several weeks of investigation by the audit firm, it was determined that the accounts receivable balances on the hospital's balance sheet were severely overstated. Nine months previously, as receivables deteriorated and the hospital ran short of cash, the chief financial officer had stopped making required payroll tax deposits. By the time the IRS became involved, over $1 million in payroll taxes were overdue.

Incredulous board members learned that the IRS was considering seizing their personal assets to satisfy the hospital's obligations. Immediately, more than one-third of the board resigned. A hastily arranged loan was approved to satisfy the tax obligations. Both the chief executive and chief financial officer were fired.

This board learned a very hard lesson. When the chief financial officer wants to conceal a major problem, it is possible to do it in spite of the annual review process. Special reports, such as testing the integrity of accounts receivable, are absolutely necessary to provide additional assurance to the board about the organization's financial status. Unfortunately for this hospital, it was too late. The hospital was sold to avoid filing for bankruptcy. The board members kept their personal assets. Perhaps they would be more inquisitive about their organization's financial statements if their cars, homes, and other personal assets were at risk if they did not do a thorough enough job.

The annual audit should include traditional reports such as the opinion letter, financial statements, and the management letter. Additional communication expectations should be articulated, a mid-year follow-up review should be required, and one or more special analysis projects should be included in the request for proposal (RFP) to ensure that major problem areas receive more than the minimum review required by generally accepted accounting practices. A sample RFP for audit services incorporating all of these elements is provided in Appendix E at the end of this book. Once the scope of the engagement is finalized, the organization can focus its efforts on selecting the best financial auditor.

SELECTING THE BEST AUDITOR

Audit services should be subjected to the RFP process at least every five years, even if the current audit firm is doing a good job. The learning curve involved makes changing auditors annually inadvisable. However, keeping the same auditors for a decade or more without periodically evaluating the competition is equally inadvisable. A well-designed RFP is the first step in selecting the best auditor. But what are the most critical aspects of the process? As with other types of consultants, they are interviews and reference checks.

All three types of accounting firms, whether "big five," specialty, or local, assign a team of accountants to healthcare organization audits. The teams usually comprise junior accountants, mid-level accountants, and an engagement leader. Junior accountants are usually assigned data gathering and routine testing assignments. Mid-level accountants often coordinate the audit and interface with the organization's accounting staff. The engagement leader, usually a partner in the accounting firm, interacts with senior management and approves the work of junior and mid-level accountants. The engagement leader is by far the most critical member of the financial audit team, and he or she should be interviewed and have his or her references thoroughly checked. The chief executive, chief financial officer, and the chairman of the board's finance committee should be personally involved in the interviews and reference checks. The quality of an accounting engagement is most often determined by the quality of the engagement leader, not the size of the accounting firm or the geographic scope of its practice.

What should you look for in an audit engagement leader? Ability to communicate honestly and effectively is most important. An excellent engagement leader knows he or she has an obligation to the client to make its financial position clearly understood to the governing board. Sometimes this takes great effort, since not all clients know what the right questions are or when to ask them. The excellent engagement leader says what needs to be said, without regard to the politics of the organization or the firm he or she represents.

Selecting the best auditor also entails making a definitive decision on the conflict of interest issue. It is very common today for accounting firms to perform both the audit and other consulting assignments for healthcare organizations, which can lead to an inherent and very problematic conflict. While it may seem too restrictive, accounting firms should be disqualified from all other types of consulting for the organization. Any potential reduction in the objectivity of the audit process is detrimental to the healthcare organization. There is no question that having one firm handle both audits and consulting is a major conflict of interest for the consultants. Many good accounting and consulting firms are available, so there is no need to use the same firm for both kinds of services. Therefore, while common, this practice should be eliminated completely.

Of course other RFP considerations should also be part of the selection decision. Firm references, professional fees, and timeframe to complete the audit are all important selection criteria. But in the final analysis, the quality of the engagement leader is the determining factor in selecting the best financial auditor.

EVALUATING AUDITORS

Once the audit firm is selected, the wise healthcare governing board conducts an annual evaluation of its services. The evaluation should take place following the suggested mid-year accounting review.

The finance committee of the board, working with the chief executive and chief financial officer, should perform the annual review. The first part of the review should cover the annual audit process. Questions the finance committee and senior management should ask regarding the audit include the following:

1. Was the audit performed on schedule and on budget?
2. Was the audit staff professional and thorough?
3. Were the audit results communicated effectively to management and board leaders?
4. Were audit recommendations thorough and effective?

5. Did the engagement leader help us understand our weaknesses and strengths?
6. Did the audit result in definitive improvements?

Beyond these questions, you must also determine if the engagement leader has been thoroughly honest and objective in his or her reports and recommendations. While this requires subjective judgment, it is a critical aspect of evaluating the accounting engagement. The most definitive question when reaching a decision in this area is whether management and board members trust the auditor and his or her assessment of the organization.

Scheduling the evaluation in the middle of the year, following the mid-year update to the board, enables the board and senior management to assess whether the auditor's previous recommendations are being acted upon. Some progressive boards schedule the mid-year update as an educational opportunity, requiring the auditors to provide the board with a preview of what kinds of issues and priorities the board can expect in the year ahead. The quality of these educational presentations is yet another opportunity for the board to evaluate its auditors.

PITFALLS TO AVOID WITH AUDITORS

The easiest pitfall to avoid is failing to evaluate or reevaluate the scope of services provided by the current or competitive audit firms. Audit services should be treated like any other ongoing consulting service: they should be periodically evaluated for quality, cost effectiveness, and service to the organization.

Another common pitfall that governing boards should avoid is delegating the selection of the audit firm and ongoing communication with the firm exclusively to senior management. Audit firms should be retained by and report to the governing board. There should be regular direct communication between board leaders and the audit firm. There should also be opportunities for board leaders to request and receive objective feedback about the performance of senior management. However, it is not the responsibility of audit firms to advise the board on the merits of retaining or separating members of management. That responsibility rests exclusively with the board.

The typical once-a-year report from the audit firm should be avoided in favor of at least two reports per year to the board. The first report should take place at the time of the annual financial audit. The second report should take place approximately six months later and include a progress report on how management is following up on identified problems and financial performance weaknesses.

Governing boards should not passively receive reports from their audit firms. It is not uncommon, even for financially distressed organizations, for a board to receive a financial audit showing dismal performance but to have no questions. Governing boards should always be prepared to question the audit firm, regardless of the year's results, but especially if the results are negative.

Finally, governing boards should avoid any conflicts of interest in the selection and retention of audit consultants. Conflicts of interest diminish the objectivity of the annual audit and must be avoided or else the objectivity necessary from an independent auditor may not be received. If the auditors seek additional professional fees for consulting projects, their independence is likely to be severely compromised.

CHECKLIST FOR SUCCESSFUL AUDIT REVIEWS

Receiving honest and objective annual audit reviews is an absolute necessity for any healthcare organization. Governing boards of failed hospitals and healthcare systems have understood in hindsight that their organization's downfall was aided by lack of knowledgeable questions being asked by members of the board and less than forthright audit reviews.

Audit consultants should not assume that their healthcare clients are mind readers. On the other hand, governing boards and senior management must seek the very best audit advisors and work hard to preserve their independence. Five keys ensure success in achieving successful audit reviews:

1. *Select.* Select the best possible engagement leader and be willing to listen carefully to what he or she says about the organization.
2. *Question.* Be prepared to ask probing questions to ensure that the knowledge gained during the audit process is accurately communicated to the board and management.

3. *Avoid.* Avoid potential conflicts of interest completely by not allowing audit consultants to perform other types of consulting services for management.
4. *Augment.* Don't be satisfied with a standard audit. Periodically add special analysis reports of key areas to ensure that the organization is not limiting the scope of accounting reviews to minimum requirements.
5. *Evaluate.* Evaluate the performance of audit firms annually and conduct a thorough RFP process at least every five years.

CONCLUSION

By selecting the best accounting firm, questioning the results of an audit, augmenting the review with special analyses, and evaluating the performance of the accounting firm, the governing board is fulfilling its responsibilities of financial oversight. If the board does not perform these responsibilities well, it may find itself requiring the services of the most expensive and intrusive consultants in the healthcare industry. Turnaround consultants are considered in the next chapter.

CHAPTER EIGHT

Turnaround Consultants

I F A T U R N A R O U N D consultant is needed, the governing board has failed in its responsibilities. The board is ultimately responsible for its organization, for better or for worse. When a turnaround consultant is necessary, the governing board should accept full responsibility, and its leaders should resign. New leadership will be sorely required if the organization is to survive.

I wrote the first healthcare industry book on turnarounds. *Managing a Hospital Turnaround* was largely a case study on how one financially distressed community hospital was turned around using "back to basics" ideas. After its publication in the 1990s, a consulting discipline emerged that focused on turnarounds. Many consulting practices and turnaround management companies were established and are thriving today. Even big accounting firms and established management consulting companies started or invested in healthcare turnaround divisions. Rather than declining in the new millennium, these firms seem to be gaining momentum as even more healthcare organizations lapse into financial disaster. Turnarounds are a growth business for consultants. How sad for our healthcare industry.

After providing turnaround consulting and interim chief executive officer services to highly distressed healthcare organizations throughout the country, I have reached the conclusion that turnarounds represent failure far more than they represent success. While turnaround chief executives are heralded with magazine cover stories and healthcare industry accolades, the very nature of a turnaround speaks more to the failure of leadership that preceded the turnaround than the accomplishment of leadership when a turnaround is successful and widely heralded.

The governing board is primarily responsible for the failure of leadership. Every healthcare organization that experiences acute financial distress had warning signs that were ignored or handled ineptly by its governing board. When an organization becomes so troubled that a turnaround is necessary, it usually has a multi-year track record of decline followed by a catastrophic financial event.

When the catastrophic event occurs, the board typically fires the chief executive officer and then conducts a hurried and superficial search for a turnaround consultant to save the organization. Or the board hires the first unemployed chief executive it finds who talks big and works cheap. Ironically, many turnaround consulting firms have earned the well-deserved reputation of doing everything but saving the organization. A turnaround may morph into a sale, merger, closure, or even bankruptcy. With the help of turnaround consultants, the board of a failed organization convinces itself that the sad end of their organization was not its fault. It was the government or competition or incompetent management—anyone's fault but the board's. Both the consultants and the board members are deluding themselves.

When an organization reaches the point where a turnaround is required, that failure rests squarely with the board. If, even after retaining a turnaround consultant, the organization ultimately fails, then that, too, is the responsibility of the board. But what is a board to do if the organization's financial position becomes so distressed that it can no longer lead? Regardless of where the fault for failure rests at that point, turnaround consultants may be the only viable choice for the board.

WHEN A TURNAROUND CONSULTANT IS NECESSARY

When healthcare organizations become financially distressed, usually over a period of years, a chemical battle is waged in the brains of board members. On one front, endorphins battle for control, seeking to make the board member feel better in spite of the sorry state of the organization. On the other front, adrenaline battles for control, seeking to blame and punish someone for getting the organization into trouble in the first place. Typically, endorphins win the battle until a seminal event occurs and then adrenaline takes over. Board members go passively along for years, receiving bad news and not responding. Then they react too aggressively and without proper thought when adrenaline takes over.

Seminal events come in several forms. When financial losses mount, a board may face the prospect of not meeting lending covenants. If finances deteriorate even further, ongoing obligations cannot be met when cash is exhausted. At other times, chief executives quit or are fired. If any of these untoward events occur, a turnaround consultant may become absolutely necessary.

It is an odd coincidence that a turnaround is sometimes preceded by a major investment or facility upgrade generated by past success and a desire to make major improvements for the organization's future. It is ironic that the optimistic financial projections necessary to float bond issues become the undoing of the management team who prepared them (often with the assistance of overly optimistic financial consultants). Sometimes it seems that the "field of dreams" theory—if we build it, they will come—is being practiced when these optimistic ventures fail to achieve their goals.

New Hospital, Old Problems: Tremendous excitement surrounded the building of a completely new hospital facility and attached physician medical center in a suburban community. In a bold move, the hospital board approved borrowing nearly $100 million to build a new hospital on a strategically located site five miles from the old hospital. The community was located in one of the fastest growing counties in the state, and the old hospital could not accommodate the influx of new patients and new doctors.

The hospital had never been a good financial performer; however, it routinely covered losses by active fund-raising programs. Its growing community enabled it to project profitable financial operations in the future by accommodating its growing population and by joining forces with its physicians in a wholly hospital-owned physician practice subsidiary. It seemed to the board, management, and medical staff that the new hospital would be wildly successful.

After the new hospital was built, the situation became wild, but not in the way imagined. To avoid angering the downtown community, the hospital kept the old building open after it relocated most services to the new facility, thereby eliminating some projected savings. When 70 physicians became salaried employees at the new hospital, their productivity plummeted, and the economics of the newly formed joint venture became adversarial.

After only one year of operation, the hospital teetered on the verge of bankruptcy. The board blamed the chief executive and fired him. A turnaround firm was quickly retained and concluded the board itself had made many poor decisions in the years leading up to the catastrophe. The board, however, refused to admit any shortcomings and refused to make any changes in governance. The turnaround consultant soon resigned. This shocked the board into action. They rehired the consultant who was then able to supervise necessary governance changes and work successfully with the new board to achieve the turnaround. The arrogance of the original board and the ineptness of management nearly ruined the first new hospital built in the area in thirty years.

Less common than financial distress is quality of care and employee distress. Severe quality problems may come to light through accreditation or regulatory inspections. Quality problems may also come to light through malpractice cases and high-profile medical mishaps. Employee-related distress may evolve when employees unionize or strike because of concerns about working conditions. These nonfinancial kinds of distress may also necessitate a turnaround consultant.

A failed search for a chief executive may also trigger the need for a turnaround consultant. If the search cannot be completed because the organization is so troubled it cannot attract a quality chief executive officer, then fundamental problems exist that need to be fixed before the chief executive search can be restarted.

A turnaround consultant is needed whenever there is a leadership vacuum at the organization. This vacuum may occur because the leadership is incompetent or absent. Regardless of the reason, when leadership is lacking in distressed organizations, it must be compensated for by experts. Enter the turnaround consultant.

DEFINING THE ENGAGEMENT SCOPE

When a governing board makes the decision that a turnaround consultant is necessary, the next challenge is to carefully define what is needed from the consultant. The first step in defining the scope is to define the end point or objective of the consultation. In other words, what must be accomplished to define the turnaround consultation as a success? The end point can be defined in several different ways. The organization may designate desired financial targets. For an organization losing money on operations, the objective could be returning to a desired level of profitability. Another option is to define the endpoint in terms of leadership; for example, recruiting a new chief executive officer along with a new governing board. Yet another end point could be the successful sale or merger of the organization, although some might argue that this option does not represent a true turnaround.

Once the end point is established, defining what the turnaround firm should accomplish comes next. There are four elements to a successful turnaround consulting engagement. First, turnaround leadership must be established. Usually this means an interim chief executive officer experienced in running distressed healthcare organizations. In some cases, the turnaround consultant may replace other senior management positions on a temporary basis.

Next, the turnaround firm should also be made accountable for performance milestones in the scope of the engagement. Monthly or quarterly targets should be established throughout the engagement. Although rarely done, the turnaround firm should also evaluate and prepare to make restructuring decisions about the board itself.

Every distressed organization has a dysfunctional board. Therefore, turnaround firms should always be required to critically evaluate and make changes in the board. At a minimum, the board chairman must step down at the beginning of a turnaround. This is a positive signal that change in the organization will begin with the board. Sometimes it is necessary to replace all or most of the board members and start over.

Finally, the scope of the engagement should specify a timeframe. Nowhere in healthcare consulting is a time limit more applicable than a turnaround. One year should be the maximum allowable time for any turnaround consultation.

SELECTING THE BEST TURNAROUND CONSULTANT

After determining the scope of the engagement, the next challenge is selecting the best turnaround consultant. Fortunately, a wide range of choices exists. Several large healthcare management companies have turnaround divisions that offer consulting, including turnaround management services. In addition, a number of medium-size specialty firms offer turnaround management consulting services. Finally, several small firms offer turnaround services to healthcare clients. Most firms provide their turnaround consulting services nationally.

Three decisive factors should be considered when hiring a turnaround consultant. First, the firm should have current experience in turning around distressed organizations. Some firms presenting themselves as experts have little or no experience of successful turnarounds. Checking references with former clients is extremely important in the selection process. The turnaround should have been performed at least one year previously.

The second important factor is the turnaround leader. While the turnaround firm itself may be top notch, if the turnaround leader for the engagement is inexperienced or incompetent, the turnaround will probably fail. The importance of experience applies to both the firm and the turnaround leader.

Finally, the leadership style is critically important. Many interim turnaround leaders have earned the reputation of "slash and burn" leaders because they inevitably institute large-scale staff layoffs and service cutbacks. This type of leadership may work for a brief period, but few if any organizations regain their strength with a "slasher" at the helm. You should seek a turnaround firm and leader who can help rebuild the organization, not accelerate its decline.

Price considerations are also important when selecting a turnaround consultant. You should be willing to pay top professional fees for top turnaround advice and leadership. As with other kinds of consulting, if the price is low, there is usually a good reason: experience or success may be lacking. On the other hand, paying top dollar does not ensure success. The board must work hard to determine that it is spending its turnaround dollars wisely.

PREREQUISITES FOR A SUCCESSFUL OUTCOME

The success of any turnaround begins with the governing board. The board initiates the process by selecting a qualified turnaround consultant and carefully defining the scope of expectations for the consultant. The first priority of the turnaround consultant should be to assess the board itself and determine what governance weaknesses must be addressed. The essential first step in improving governance is changing board leadership. It is neither fair nor wise for the board to merely fire the chief executive officer and bring in a turnaround consultant when things go terribly wrong. The board itself, especially the chair, should leave office. This paves the way for new leadership to begin making necessary changes at the top of the troubled organization.

In addition to its leadership, the entire governing board membership and its policies and procedures should be thoroughly examined and improved. A prerequisite for success in a turnaround situation is the board's willingness to make changes in governance to correct past failures before the difficult work begins to improve the rest of the organization.

Another prerequisite of success is a board willing to facilitate change throughout the organization to correct what went wrong to place the organization in jeopardy. The turnaround consultant must have the support of the board to make necessary changes at all levels of the organization. There can be no "sacred cows" if the organization is to recover.

The Second Time Around: It may take more than one turnaround before the governing board gets the message. In one such instance, a hospital experienced severe financial distress in the early 1990s. The chief executive retired and the board retained a turnaround consultant. After nearly a year of cost cutting, program curtailments, and service reductions, costs had been reduced enough to stabilize the hospital's deteriorating finances. A new chief executive was hired, and everyone breathed a sigh of relief.

The new chief executive energized the previously troubled hospital and within a short time a new strategic plan was in place, money was in the bank again, and employee and physician morale was restored. The hospital and chief executive even won industry accolades for the dramatic turnaround. Things went wonderfully for nearly five years. Everything had changed and improved. Except the governing board.

Six years after the turnaround the hospital's finances began deteriorating again. The next year, things got worse. By the third year, the hospital was more financially distressed than it had been during the period preceding its first turnaround. The chief executive convinced the board that everything would get better soon. They believed him. Unfortunately, he was wrong.

During the fourth year, the hospital ran out of cash. The chief executive was fired, and the turnaround consultant was invited back to start all over again. He refused to accept the offer until the board chairman agreed to step down. After a prolonged battle, the board chairman resigned. It took two years for the hospital to fully emerge from its near failure, but this time something even more dramatic occurred. The board completely reorganized itself, appointed new officers, recruited new members, and created a comprehensive set of governance policies designed to avoid the disaster that had occurred not once, but twice.

It takes great courage and conviction to initiate and facilitate change in a troubled organization. The process begins with the board. To be successful, the board must keep the end point in mind. It should envision a day when the organization is recovering and turnaround consultants are no longer needed. Fostering the changes necessary in the organization and board and recruiting permanent new leadership is a major factor in making that day arrive. The board must transform its shortcomings into strengths to recruit its new chief executive officer.

PITFALLS TO AVOID WITH TURNAROUND CONSULTANTS

There are numerous pitfalls in turnaround consultation. First and foremost is superficially evaluating alternatives and selecting a consultant arbitrarily. A governing board may sit passively through years of declining performance, taking little or no corrective action. When the moment of truth arrives and it becomes painfully clear that the organization is seriously troubled, that same passive board will often make an instantaneous decision when selecting a turnaround consultant. Both the passive approach and the instant call to arms are wrong. A board should deliberately evaluate at least three or four alternatives with a thorough RFP and interview process and select the best turnaround consultant. While this may take discipline when it seems the organization is falling apart, it is the right approach.

Another pitfall to avoid when selecting a turnaround consultant is relying on the reputation of the firm without giving enough consideration to who the firm is sending to perform the turnaround. The success of turnaround work rests with its leadership, and the onsite leader is the most important element of bringing that leadership to the troubled organization. While the firm's reputation is important, the skill and experience of the onsite leader are more critical.

When the turnaround is underway, another pitfall that should be avoided is firing all of top management and replacing them with interim executives. This can be very destructive and expensive. Some firms automatically use this approach as a method of increasing their professional fees and the organization's dependence on the turnaround firm. This should be resisted because it guarantees two complete senior management changes. The first occurs during the turnaround. The second one occurs when the permanent chief executive is hired and replaces the interim executives with his or her own team. This double turnover at the top is always disruptive and often unnecessary.

Another pitfall to avoid with turnaround firms is becoming too dependent on them. Some boards have a tendency to over-rely on their consultants, at the expense of completing the turnaround and securing new permanent leadership. Turnaround teams are simply not effective at overseeing institutions on a long-term basis, no matter how bad the problems are. Turnarounds should have a definite timeframe not exceeding one year. All boards that retain turnaround consultants should have an exit strategy and an exit timeframe. Boards should also take care not to set too low a threshold for turnaround success. It is common for a financially distressed healthcare organization to declare victory when the organization's finances break even. Breaking even is just a milestone on the journey to financial stability. It should never be an end point.

CHECKLIST FOR A SUCCESSFUL TURNAROUND EXPERIENCE

Avoiding all of the pitfalls associated with turnaround consultants comes down to simple strategies. Suggestions for a successful experience include the following six steps.

1. *Avoid.* Try to avoid the circumstances that require turnarounds.
2. *Decide.* Decide whether a turnaround is the desired outcome. If the board wants to sell or merge with another organization, it may be best to go straight to that strategy.
3. *Hire.* If a turnaround is desired or needed, the best turnaround advisor should be selected. Pay whatever it takes to hire the best.

4. *Change.* The critical first step in any turnaround process is to change the board by replacing the chairman, recruiting new and better members, and writing—and then living up to—governance policies that ensure turnaround consultation will never be needed again.
5. *Conclude.* Once started, the turnaround should proceed promptly. Unless a compelling reason is present, turnarounds should be concluded in a year or less.
6. *Commit.* Make sure that a turnaround is the last one ever needed. Start a new post-turnaround era with a new board, new leadership, and a new commitment to act *before* disaster strikes.

CONCLUSION

The very best healthcare turnaround is one that is avoided before it begins. Many consultants are available to work collaboratively with management and the board to improve the organization's performance. If you have the choice, and you do in most cases, one of these consultants should be retained to work with management and the board before problems become so severe that turnaround consultants are the only viable option. In most cases, management and the board working diligently together can resolve even the most difficult problems. If ongoing problems are not resolved, then it may be time for the board to consider recruiting a new chief executive, the subject of the next chapter.

CHAPTER NINE

Chief Executive Officer Search

FOR A HEALTHCARE organization that is about to undertake the search for a new chief executive officer (CEO), the stakes are high. Many searches are doomed from the start because of a dysfunctional board. Other searches are bungled when the overriding desire to complete the search quickly undermines the quality of the search process. Searching for the right chief executive officer is actually a marketing challenge for the board. Like any other marketing challenge, a good product or chief executive opportunity must exist before it can be sold to the best-qualified candidate.

The selection of a new chief executive officer is a defining moment for any healthcare organization. The search process may be handled by the organization's board, delegated to an executive search firm, or a combination of both approaches may be used. A key factor in deciding which approach will produce optimum results is the amount of time and expertise a board has to invest in the search process.

An important preliminary to the search is a careful review of the reason for the chief executive opening. If the current chief executive is retiring after a distinguished twenty-year tenure, the search for a replacement is straightforward. Alternately, if the chief executive was terminated after experiencing tenure of less than five years, the chief executive search process and the timing of when to start it may be more complicated.

The search for a new chief executive, regardless of the reason for the vacancy, is the most important job of a healthcare organization's board. It requires quality time to perform the job well, regardless of whether a consultant is retained to help. This period of leadership transition is also a remarkably good time for the board to take stock of its own and the chief executive officer's responsibilities. If there ever was a time for improving governance effectiveness and refining the expectations for the chief executive position, this is it.

A chief executive officer vacancy creates a great opportunity, as well as considerable anxiety. Boards often rush to fill the position when a more deliberate process is in the organization's best long-term interests. Recruiting the very best new chief executive should be the ultimate goal, not the speed of filling the vacancy. Boards should tolerate some of the uncertainty that can come with a chief executive position vacancy rather than move too fast to fill it and later regret a hasty decision.

Consultants can assist boards with the chief executive officer search process. A traditional retained search, with an executive search firm performing most of the search process guided by the board, is right for some chief executive recruitments. A facilitated search in which the consultant provides overall direction to the board as it performs most of the search tasks is also a viable option. In some circumstances, the board may be qualified to perform the chief executive search itself without any consulting assistance. Deciding which approach to use is the first challenge. Highlighting the merits of various search approaches and helping the board select the best approach for their needs are the goals of this chapter.

WHEN TO RETAIN AN EXECUTIVE SEARCH CONSULTANT

A board with advance warning of an impending chief executive vacancy is more likely to be able to perform the search itself or utilize only minimal consulting assistance in the form of a facilitated search. If the incumbent chief executive is planning to retire in the coming year, and several senior executives are clearly qualified and interested in the position, the board may want to consider an abbreviated search process to interview the internal candidates and select the best successor. Most executive search consultants resist this approach, insisting that a full-scope executive search is needed for every chief executive vacancy. Some boards may view that opinion as self-serving, choosing instead to use an abbreviated approach if both the board and the departing chief executive have done a good job with succession planning.

At the other extreme, if the board terminated the organization's third chief executive in the past four years, considerable professional consultation may be needed to objectively identify the reasons for the turnover and what needs to change before selecting a new chief executive officer who will perform as needed and stay in the position for at least five years.

If the organization is experiencing excessive chief executive turnover, either through terminations or resignations, the board must resolve the turnover problems before starting the next chief executive search. Naming an internal executive as interim chief executive or retaining an interim chief executive from outside the organization may be just what is needed to allow time to thoroughly assess the reasons for past turnover. Boards should never feel compelled to fill an open chief executive officer position immediately, especially if the board itself may be partially to blame for the vacancy.

If chief executive turnover is a problem, consultation is always advisable. Before starting a search, the consultant should work closely with the board to identify and rectify the problems that have led to excessive turnover. Only then can the next chief executive search produce optimum results.

DEFINING THE ENGAGEMENT SCOPE

Time, expertise, and money are key factors in deciding whether to retain an executive search consultant. If the board has the time (that is, adequate notice of upcoming turnover) and the expertise (directors with previous experience in searches), conducting the search without professional assistance should be considered. If the board has neither the time nor the expertise to perform the search itself, then it will have to invest in an appropriately qualified consultant to assist in the search. If the facilitated approach is used, the investment in consulting fees will be modest. If a traditional retained search is used, the fees will be more substantial, but worth it if the right new chief executive is successfully recruited.

In the facilitated search approach, the consultant:

- helps the board define its expectations for the new chief executive officer, articulate the specifications for qualified candidates, and establish a CEO search committee;

- advises the CEO search committee on how to "source" candidates for the position, using direct mail, professional association contacts, ads in professional journals, internet sites, and so forth;
- assists the search committee with approaches and questions for reference checks and preliminary interviews with candidates;
- advises the search committee on selecting three to five finalists;
- participates in the interviews with finalists and advises the search committee on final selection; and
- assists the search committee with "deal closing" activities such as contract negotiation, transition planning, and so forth.

In each activity, the search consultant is acting as an advisor to the search committee, which will do the actual work of sorting through candidates' resumes or CVs, conducting initial interviews, and organizing the process for final interviews and chief executive officer selection. Undertaking a facilitated search approach requires a search committee with the time to perform these tasks competently. Many boards possess the expertise, that, when coupled with excellent consulting advice, can enable them to conduct an excellent chief executive search.

In a traditional retained search for a new chief executive officer, the consultant:

- drafts or updates the position description and job specifications;
- identifies all interested and qualified candidates;
- screens interested candidates through phone and preliminary personal interviews;
- evaluates and selects ten to fifteen candidates for review with the search committee;
- assists the search committee with selecting three to five finalists for interviews and performs reference checks; and
- assists the search committee with "deal closing" activities such as contract negotiation, transition planning, and so forth.

In each of these activities, the search consultant acts on behalf of the search committee up until the final selection of the first-choice candidate. This approach works well when the search committee's time is limited, because it allows them to focus on selecting among qualified candidates rather than finding those candidates.

Professional fees for the two consulting approaches are quite different. A facilitated approach will result in consulting fees of approximately 10 to 20 percent of the new chief executive's base salary. The retained search approach will result in professional fees of approximately 30 to 40 percent of the chief executive's base salary. In both cases, consulting firms will also charge the client for out-of-pocket expenses such as telephone, mail, travel, and report preparation.

The facilitated search approach is far less common than the retained search approach. Traditional retained search firms may resist the facilitated approach because of lower fees, underutilization of their full resource capabilities, or lack of complete control of the search process. Boards should consider doing the search themselves or using the facilitated approach more often than is currently the practice. Good boards can perform a chief executive search effectively, and no consulting firm will ever have as much to gain, or to lose, by the process as the board itself.

SELECTING THE BEST CHIEF EXECUTIVE SEARCH ADVISOR

Experience in successful chief executive officer searches is the single most important factor in selecting the best search advisor. A successful search is one where the chief executive serves for at least five years and meets or exceeds the expectations of his or her board.

Performing chief executive searches for similar organizations should be a prerequisite in selecting a consultant. If the board is filling the chief executive position of a small rural hospital, a search consultant whose work focuses primarily on large urban medical centers should not be a strong contender. Likewise, the board of a suburban hospital that is part of a multi-hospital system should not select a search consultant who specializes in searches for small independent rural hospitals.

It is not enough for a consultant to simply have performed chief executive searches. A board must retain a consultant whose searches actually worked for both chief executive and hospital. Tenure in position following the search is a good indicator of success. If the chief executive stays for five or more years, it is likely that both the chief executive and his or her board have been well satisfied with the search results. If, on the other hand, the search consultant rarely places a chief executive who stays for five years, it may be indicate quality problems with the consultant.

A consultant who does not fully understand the organization will not be able to find the type of candidates that meets its needs. Just as important is the failure to work successfully with an organization to address internal problems before starting a chief executive search. If a search consultant cannot help a dysfunctional board or organization improve before initiating a chief executive search, then the client is unlikely to attract a quality chief executive.

What can you do to ensure you are retaining the very best chief executive search consultant? Reference checking is the most important tool available. Prospective search consultants should be able to demonstrate that they have successfully performed chief executive searches for at least five similar organizations that have retained their chief executives for five or more years. In selection of search consultants, use of old (three to five years previous) references is more important than current references. Consultants or consulting firms lacking this level of successful experience should not be considered for chief executive officer searches.

In addition to reference checking, "chemistry" between the consultant and the board and organization leaders is also an important factor. A chief executive officer search involves having the search consultant represent the organization to prospective candidates. The board should be assured through personal interviews that a consultant who will represent the organization positively to chief executive candidates is selected. The board should also be interested in selecting a consultant who listens well, both to the board and to its candidates.

In selecting the best consultant, first narrow the field to those with experience and an excellent track record. Then, among this group of pre-qualified consultants, select the one who will represent the organization well. Experience and trust—never select a search consultant unless both of these criteria are met. An RFP process should be used to evaluate three to five search consultants. After the consultant is retained, the board needs to devote the time necessary to get the search off to a good start.

PREPARING FOR A SUCCESSFUL CHIEF EXECUTIVE SEARCH

It is said that success in business is 80 percent perspiration and 20 percent inspiration. It may also be said that success in a chief executive search is 80 percent preparation. This is true regardless of whether the board conducts the search itself or retains a consulting firm to conduct a facilitated or retained search. A good place to start preparing for the search is with the board.

Before starting the chief executive officer search, the board should assess its own strengths and weaknesses. First and foremost, this assessment should entail a candid review of the tenure of past chief executives. If the board has experienced excellent tenure (five years or more) from its chief executives, this is a major strength of the organization. On the other hand, if chief executives are coming and going every two or three years, then the board or the organization may have fundamental problems that need attention before another search begins. It is common for some dysfunctional organizations to experience excessive chief executive turnover due to problems with the governing board itself. Conflicts of interest, meddling in operations, and excessive attention to placating politically connected physicians are just a few of the many governance problems that lead to chief executive turnover.

> **Revolving Door CEOs:** A rural community hospital experienced an extremely high level of chief executive turnover—its past five executives averaged only two years in their positions. The board never used search consultants, expressing the collective opinion that consultants were a waste of money.
>
> After each chief executive turnover, the hospital's financial performance declined. Chief executives came and went, and employees joked in private that a revolving door should be installed in the administrator's officer. Employees and physicians were demoralized and patients began driving to the hospital 20 miles down the road, further depressing the hospital's future prospects.
>
> After the fifth chief executive's departure in ten years, the board finally decided to retain an executive search firm. The consultant assigned to the search was very experienced and quickly determined that low salary was the culprit for past chief executive turnover. He presented a "reality check" to members of the board about the appropriate compensation for recruiting and, more importantly, retaining an excellent chief executive. Although the board balked at first, the search consultant was patient and helped the board understand its role in structuring a fair market compensation plan.

Upon resolving this controversial issue, the board and search consultant worked together to perform a successful search, hiring an enthusiastic new chief executive. The chief executive served for a distinguished five years before moving on to a larger hospital. During his tenure, the hospital reestablished itself as the local healthcare provider of choice and established a firm foundation for future success.

Experienced search advisors can assist boards in pinpointing their weaknesses and correcting them before the start of a search. If the board chooses not to correct its problems, the consultant should resign because the board will be wasting the time and capability of a good search consultant. If the board is rotten, not even the most brilliant search consultant can succeed because a good chief executive candidate will sense the problems and withdraw from the search. In the unlikely event that a good candidate takes a chief executive position with a bad board, the candidate will soon resign over matters of principal or be fired for "doing the right thing," starting the chief executive officer search process all over again.

After assessing itself and correcting any fundamental governance problems, the board should next assess the strengths and weaknesses of the chief executive officer position and its expectations for the new chief executive. A chief executive vacancy is an excellent opportunity to review and update the job description, compensation and benefits, and the desired personal and professional attributes required in a new chief executive. It is also an opportune time for the board to articulate short- and long-term goals for the new chief executive.

MARKETING THE ORGANIZATION

When the board and chief executive position assessments have been completed, it is time to focus on marketing strategy. A good chief executive officer search is, at its core, a marketing challenge. An enlightened board views the search as an opportunity to present the organization, community, and future aspirations of the organization in a fashion that will attract the best and brightest candidates. If the organization is marketed successfully during the search process, there will be a number of very well-qualified candidates from which to choose the next chief executive. On the other hand, if the organization is not marketed positively, the pool of qualified and interested candidates will be small or nonexistent, no matter what approach is used to perform the search.

How should the organization prepare to market itself? First, a high-quality packet of background material for prospective candidates should be assembled. This packet should contain recent annual reports, current strategic plans, audited financial statements, publications, organization charts, lists of governing board members and management staff, and committee lists for the clinical staff. In addition, local public relations material should be added to show the community in the most positive light.

The marketing process also includes preparing to interview prospective candidates. Travel agents, hotel accommodations, and local transportation arrangements should be prearranged and ready to use with prospective candidates. Arrangements for community tours for candidates and their spouses, promoting the most positive aspects of the community while being careful to point out the community's weaknesses, should be finalized. Advance preparation makes it possible to impress candidates and to present a consistent perspective to all candidates who make it to the interview phase of the search.

Finally, marketing the organization involves providing references on the organization itself. When the chief executive search reaches the final phases, it is just as important for the board to provide references as it is to check references for the candidates. The most thorough candidates will ask for references from the audit firm, lead legal counsel, community leaders, and perhaps even past chief executives. The board should welcome this request and should give advance thought to who can provide thorough and positive references. If the board cannot identify any such positive references, it needs to go back to the governance assessment process and revisit its own performance. A questionable reference from someone such as the audit partner, legal counsel, or community leader is the last thing the number one choice for the chief executive position needs to hear.

When board and chief executive position assessments are complete and advance preparation steps for marketing the organization are completed, then and only then is the board ready to begin the chief executive officer search by naming a search committee. The reward for all this advance preparation will be a smoother search and an organization that candidates recognize as having its act together. This recognition is the first step in attracting the best chief executive candidates.

DECISION TO DELEGATE

Hiring a new chief executive is one of the most important responsibilities of a governing board. Importance notwithstanding, it is not practical for the entire board to conduct the chief executive search. Some delegation is absolutely necessary. It is common for a board to designate a chief executive search committee made up of members of the board and clinical staff leaders and occasionally additional members from interested outside constituencies such as local business and community leaders. An effective search committee is given the important responsibility of recommending a final candidate or slate of candidates to the full governing board for approval.

The search committee may do the search itself or it may use a facilitated or retained search consultant approach to discharge its responsibility. If a consultant is used, the search committee conducts the consultant selection. The search committee's primary job, whether or not assisted by a consultant, is to attract applications, screen the applicants, interview the best candidates, and make a preliminary selection of the finalist candidates for subsequent presentation to the full board.

Certain tasks during the search should not be delegated by the search committee if a search consultant is used, including marketing the organization. Advance preparation of background materials by the organization is the first opportunity for marketing, and the best materials should be assembled by the organization. Members of the search committee or people within the organization that the committee designates should handle marketing the community and the organization. A consultant cannot market them successfully.

Nor should narrowing down the universe of applicants be entirely delegated to search consultants. If a chief executive position attracts one hundred applicants, search consultants can apply the organization's search criteria to select the best 10 percent. However, the search committee should be involved in selecting the best candidates for on-site interviews. For example, if five candidates will be interviewed, the search committee should be involved in the narrowing process that picks the top 5 of the best 10 applicants.

After the initial interviews, the search committee should not delegate the task of picking the two or three candidates who are selected for second interviews. Nor should the search committee delegate the entire responsibility of conducting reference checks to the search consultant. Even if the consultant has performed preliminary reference checks of finalists, members of the search committee should personally conduct the final reference checks.

After final interviews have been conducted and references checked, the search committee should select its first-choice candidate. While feedback and suggestions from consultants are important, the search committee should make the choice of the best candidate to recommend to the full board. It is not uncommon for the full board to conduct a third interview before proceeding with approval of the finalist candidate as the new chief executive.

Finally, the search committee should select one of its members to negotiate the contract with the first-choice candidate. When the contract is signed, the appropriate internal and external announcements can be prepared and the transition to the organization's new chief executive officer initiated.

PITFALLS TO AVOID IN CHIEF EXECUTIVE SEARCHES

The greatest pitfall for a governing board to avoid is beginning a chief executive officer search when known governance problems are unresolved. A board that does not have its own house in order cannot perform a successful search, even if an excellent consultant is retained to assist. Related to this pitfall is absence of candor. A board that cannot be honest in assessing its strengths and weaknesses cannot perform a successful search. The best candidates will discover the board's problems and lack of candor during the search and drop out, leaving only the less-qualified candidates.

> **Terminal Conflict:** A large urban hospital was experiencing extreme financial distress when it fired its chief executive. The hospital was completely demoralized, having fallen into near-bankruptcy from the position it had held as an award-winning institution several years before.
>
> An interim chief executive was hired to stabilize the hospital, and a consultant was retained to provide guidance to the interim chief executive and board and to conduct the search for a permanent chief executive officer. The consultant evaluated the governing board and found it to be performing its duties poorly. The board had failed to act promptly when the hospital's finances began to decline and failed to address significant

problems of medical quality. In addition, the consultant determined that the board chair was involved in a severe conflict of interest as an associate in a professional firm that received hundreds of thousands of dollars per year for its services to the hospital.

The consultant confronted the board with its shortcomings and refused to initiate the search until the chairman stepped down and his firm discontinued professional services. A boardroom brawl ensued that lasted for over a month. Ultimately, the chairman stepped down and later resigned from the board after the hospital severed all ties to his firm.

With new officers, a new attitude pervaded the board. They aggressively addressed long-time shortcomings in their own performance. The search for the new chief executive was begun several months later, and a very enthusiastic and capable chief executive was hired. He cited the willingness of the board to "clean up their act" as the decisive factor in attracting him to the position.

Governing boards should also avoid overdependence on search consultants who assist the search committee. Good search consultants assist governing boards; they do not act in the place of governing boards. Search committees should not delegate the critical process of narrowing down the best candidates and making the difficult choice of a final candidate.

If the search committee does use a consultant, it should consciously avoid being blinded by any particular candidate presented by a search consultant. This occurs when a search committee is presented with a group of candidates among whom only one candidate clearly meets the board's search criteria. If this situation develops, the search committee should ask the consultant to identify a new slate of candidates so that they can select the finalist from among equally qualified candidates.

Failure to thoroughly check the references of finalist candidates is another pitfall to avoid in chief executive searches. It is truly amazing that chief executives are still hired in healthcare organizations without good reference checks. Members of the search committee should personally check finalists' references and add that information to earlier reference checks performed by the search consultant.

Ideally, two or three leading candidates should reach the finalist stage. At that advanced stage in the search, the final candidates should all be qualified for the chief executive position. The challenge is selecting the finalist who can best lead the organization in the future. Sometimes each finalist is strong and no clear selection is apparent. When this happens, a major pitfall may ensue: a deadlock or strong disagreement about the first choice. To avoid this pitfall, all interested constituencies should be reminded that the board must make the ultimate selection of the chief executive. The clinical staff may prefer one candidate, the management staff may prefer another, and other interested constituencies may prefer yet a third candidate. While input is welcomed, the governing board selects the chief executive based on the recommendations of the search committee. Unanimity is desirable, but not necessarily possible in every search.

Once the chief executive is selected, a final pitfall needs to be avoided: not articulating the board's expectations of a new chief executive. Every new chief executive should have a list of short- and long-term expectations as he or she begins the new job and an evaluation process in place to determine if expectations are being met. Failure to articulate expectations nearly always results in confusion at the beginning of a new chief executive's tenure, precisely the time when clearly articulated expectations should help jump-start his or her leadership.

CHECKLIST FOR A SUCCESSFUL CHIEF EXECUTIVE SEARCH

Conducting a chief executive search is a defining moment for every governing board. Successful searches ensure the organization's future will be in good hands. Failed searches burden the organization with excessive chief executive turnover or, even worse, long tenure of a poor performer. A successful chief executive search can benefit from the selection of an effective consultant. Suggestions for a successful experience include the following six steps.

1. *Prepare.* The board should get its act together first by resolving any major governance problems and by being clear about its expectations for the chief executive position.
2. *Organize.* The board should be as involved in the search as possible. If it conducts the search itself, it should organize itself accordingly. If it retains a consultant, it should retain one with experience in chief executive searches and a track record of placements with five or more years' tenure.

3. *Market*. A well-conceived marketing strategy with assorted materials should be assembled to positively present the organization, the community, and future opportunities.
4. *Compile*. Developing a large enough candidate base to produce a very tough choice among at least three highly qualified and interested candidates at the end of the search is very important.
5. *Choose*. The board should select the strongest candidate, even if that candidate is not the first choice of some constituencies.
6. *Articulate*. Expectations must be articulated before the new chief executive starts, and the board must work collaboratively to ensure a long tenure for the most qualified chief executive candidate.

CONCLUSION

Governing boards should aspire to create an environment that will attract the best chief executive and keep that individual for at least five years. While that is not always an easy goal, the best boards strive for it. The true measure of a successful chief executive search may not be evident for several years. An excellent chief executive and an effective governing board are the essential elements of leadership needed to successfully plan for the future, the subject of the next chapter.

CHAPTER TEN

Strategic Planning

E VERY HEALTHCARE ORGANIZATION needs a sound strategic plan, but the validity of strategic planning is often questioned in today's fast-changing healthcare environment. Some say that it is impossible to plan years into the future when major shifts occur in a few brief months in the competitive market, regulatory environment, and patient utilization patterns. Is strategic planning still relevant in an era of rapid change? In a word, yes.

It is precisely because the pace of change is accelerating that healthcare organizations need a planning framework to guide strategic decisions. While planning may be more difficult in the twenty-first century, it is still a critical factor in the success of healthcare enterprises. Strategic planning may be viewed as a tremendous opportunity for an organization to reinvent itself and not only keep up with change, but use change to its best advantage.

Boards and chief executives of healthcare organizations often need help from consultants to produce the best strategic plans. Consultants can contribute a wealth of experience and insight to the process of planning for the future. Excellent consultants help leaders create a sound plan to strengthen the organization. It is imprudent for a board and executive team to embark on strategic planning without some support or input from consultants. Consultants may not have *all* the answers, but they can play a very positive role in helping the organization's leaders find the best answers in planning for their future.

What is included in a strategic plan? While healthcare organizations differ in their interpretations of what a strategic plan is, several important factors should always be present in a strategic plan:

- Environmental assessment
- Historical performance trends
- SWOT (strengths, weaknesses, opportunities, and threats) analysis
- Strategic vision statement
- Strategic goals and performance milestones
- Annual operating and capital financial projections
- Implementation plan and timetable

Why should a consultant be used for strategic planning? A competent organization could create a strategic plan using only internal resources, but the effective use of consultants can add quality and insights to a strategic plan that a completely internally developed plan may not contain. An effective strategic planning consultant adds value in two important ways: knowledge of successful and unsuccessful strategic plans of other organizations, which adds depth and experience; and an enhancement of the creative process, which yields a more effective plan.

Imagine an orchestra conductor. Truly great ones achieve success not because they are themselves virtuoso instrument performers, but because they have the talent to bring out the very best performances of a diverse group of highly talented musicians. A successful strategic planning consultant helps the organization's best thinkers produce a virtuoso performance, creating a vision for the future. While the organization may have talented individual leaders, a gifted consultant can help them achieve a collective planning performance far beyond any one individual's talents.

There are two distinct consulting approaches to strategic planning: authored and facilitated. Authored strategic planning places the primary responsibility on consultants for creating the strategic plan after considering the input and ideas of the organization's constituencies. In facilitated strategic planning, consultants guide the organization in the planning process instead of actually creating the plan. Both approaches have merits and drawbacks, and the organization must select the approach that best meets its needs. The objective of this chapter is to discuss the differences in these approaches and suggest ways to choose the best approach to meet your organization's strategic planning needs.

When is the best time to retain a strategic planning consultant and when should a strategic plan be written? All healthcare organizations should have a current strategic plan. The higher the plan's quality, the better the organization is likely to perform. Several landmark events lend themselves to the creation of a new strategic plan, including the start of a new chief executive officer's tenure. When an organization is energized by the introduction of a new leader, that leader can seize the opportunity to articulate a new vision for the organization.

A major environmental or competitive shift is another opportune time for creating a new strategic plan. If a fundamental shift occurs in the organization's marketplace, a new strategy will be needed to cope with the shift. A major upturn or downturn in the organization's performance is another ideal time to create a new strategic plan. If things are going extraordinarily well, resources may be available to accelerate the positive changes benefiting the organization. On the other hand, if key trends are declining, it may be time to rethink the organization's strategy and make changes before catastrophic declines occur.

David versus Goliath: A hospital in a small community found itself with a major competitive shift almost overnight. The governing board had been approached by a well-known health system 90 miles away with a purchase offer. The board considered and rejected the offer, assuming the system would choose another town for its next hospital acquisition. Instead, the system purchased the only other hospital in town. The competitive landscape changed immediately.

Previously, the two hospitals had split the community's healthcare business equally between them. After the acquisition, the system went to great efforts to publicize its presence in the community, highlighting the national reputation of the main hospital and clinic. The community hospital feared the health system would decimate its traditional 50 percent market share.

Instead of panicking, the hospital began a thoughtful strategic planning process. With a planning consultant acting as facilitator, it was able to identify and reinforce its strengths and to articulate its vision of the future as the "community's own hospital." Rather than directly compete with the out-of-town giant, it decided instead to focus on what it did best: primary and secondary care. The hospital created a strategic plan that reinforced its historical strengths and emphasized its local ownership and commitment to the community. Instead of trying to compete with the big-name system, it chose to invest in improving its core services. The new strategy worked. After several years, the hospital's market share improved dramatically, and its system-owned competitor began a precipitous decline, proving that good strategy can defeat hype any day.

Mergers, affiliations, and other combinations also represent optimal times for creating a new strategic plan. A new opportunity arising in the organization's marketplace should also trigger consideration of a new strategic plan. Finally, successful emergence from a period of financial distress is a good time to create a strategic plan for future success.

If it is time to develop a strategic plan, when should you consider retaining a strategic planning consultant to help? The sooner, the better. Strategic planning is one area in which a properly retained and directed consultant can make an immediate difference in the quality of a plan for the future.

DEFINING THE ENGAGEMENT SCOPE

Healthcare organization leaders embarking on strategic planning must first decide whether they want the consultant to author the plan or to facilitate the planning process. If the authored plan is chosen, a consultant or firm that can research the historical performance of the organization, its past strategies, and major internal and external trends affecting the organization must be selected. The authored approach requires consultants who can accurately and objectively assess the organization's current performance and predict future performance. It requires consultants who can identify alternative strategies for the future and select the best ones for consideration. The authored approach requires consultants with excellent written and oral communication skills.

Facilitation skills, such as the ability to ensure balanced participation in planning and brainstorming meetings, are different from the research and writing skills necessary for the authored plan approach. If strategic planning using the facilitated approach is preferred, a consultant or firm should be chosen based on their ability to facilitate and energize groups and individuals within the organization, to articulate current strengths and weaknesses, and to then brainstorm about possible future strategic directions that will best serve the organization and its constituencies. The facilitated approach also requires a consultant who can help the organization achieve consensus about desired strategies for the future. The consultant must be able to work with internal constituencies to rank and prioritize ideas, not merely identify them.

Once the planning approach that best meets the organization's needs is chosen, the scope of the engagement can be defined and selection of the best consultant to assist with strategic planning can proceed. The basic differences in scope between the authored and facilitated approaches are as follows:

Authored Strategic Plan Scope
- Research history and trends
- Identify performance trends and future projections
- Perform internal and external assessments
- Develop alternative strategies
- Recommend strategic plans

Facilitated Strategic Plan Scope
- Research history and trends
- Identify performance trends and future projections
- Assemble internal and external planning brainstorming groups
- Elicit multiple ideas and options for the future
- Develop consensus about preferred ideas
- Assemble preferred ideas into strategic plan

An authored strategic plan takes about four to six months to write with minimal involvement by the organization. A facilitated strategic plan will take approximately six to eight months to prepare, with moderate to heavy involvement by the organization. The selection of the best planning consultant is critical for success, regardless of which approach is selected.

SELECTING THE BEST PLANNING CONSULTANT

If the authored planning approach is chosen, a consultant or consulting firm with depth and multiple skills must be engaged. The initial work on an authored strategic plan requires research and historical trend projection skills. Once basic research is completed, the consulting firm must have the experience to identify the strengths and weaknesses of an organization and alternative strategies to capitalize on them. Next the consultants must have the evaluation skills to select the strategies they believe will best meet the future needs of the organization. Finally, communication skills are necessary to write a plan recommending strategies for the future. The steps of research, assessment, alternative strategies, and writing final recommendations may require different consultants or consultant teams with different skill sets, so this approach definitely lends itself to medium-size or large consulting firms.

If the facilitated approach is selected, the organization usually performs the research and trend analysis, preparing the way for a single consultant or small group of consultants to facilitate the brainstorming process. The consultant's organizational skills are used to help the client elicit ideas instead of actually authoring the ideas. The facilitation consultant should help the organization's internal constituents offer input and ideas for the future. Facilitating meetings and brainstorming sessions is the heart of the approach, which is usually longer and is sometimes "messier" than the authored approach. If the organization's leaders are soliciting ideas, and they prepare effectively, they will be besieged with strategies for the future. It takes time to process the ideas and to reach consensus on those with the most merit.

Regardless of which approach is selected, several traits are very important to look for when selecting planning consultants. The first is experience. A consultant or firm that has helped several organizations plan for the future will have insight and perspective on what is likely to work well and what is more likely to fail. Creativity is also extremely important in strategic planning. Whether the consultant is authoring the plan or facilitating brainstorming meetings, creativity is absolutely essential. The ability to challenge the organization and its status quo is a highly desirable trait for strategic planners. Some consultants have a "sixth sense" of how to challenge a client while helping its constituents think creatively. Finally, intellectual flexibility is an important characteristic. A consultant with a flexible perspective is able to stimulate an organization in a positive fashion. A consultant without flexibility usually ends up trying to convince organization leaders that there is only one way to accomplish something.

USING THE REQUEST FOR PROPOSAL EFFECTIVELY

A well-crafted request for proposal (RFP) is essential for selecting the best strategic planning consultant. The experience of the lead consultant and prior client references are two critical aspects of evaluating an RFP response. The lead consultant for a strategic plan should have all the desired traits described previously, but there is another factor that is even more important. A strategic plan, even an elegantly crafted one, is nothing more than words on paper. An effective strategic plan is one that motivates the organization to change in positive ways. When selecting a strategic planning consultant, it is vital to choose one who has a positive track record in authoring or facilitating plans that were implemented successfully. The only way to determine this is by thoroughly checking references. Several important questions should be asked when contacting references:

- Did you respect the planner?
- Did the planner help articulate a new strategic vision?
- Was the strategic planning process a success?
- Has your organization implemented the plan's strategic goals?
- Did the implementation of the plan lead the organization in a positive way?
- Would you use the same strategic planner for your next plan?

Organization leaders may want to visit the former clients of the consultant they believe is best for them as part of the reference checking process. A site visit can be invaluable in making the right choice.

After the consultants are chosen, the next challenge is preparing for a successful consultation.

PREPARING FOR A SUCCESSFUL STRATEGIC PLANNING ENGAGEMENT

Available quality time is the single most important factor in achieving a successful strategic planning engagement. Organizations that take the time to thoughtfully select a planning approach and a planning consultant must ensure that the right people have sufficient time to meaningfully participate in the strategic planning process once it begins. Quality time is important from two perspectives. First, the organization must ensure all key constituencies have time to contribute. Second, sufficient time is needed to refine strategies and ideas before they are finalized. An idea may sound great at first, but as it is discussed and fully evaluated, its flaws may become apparent. Time to fully explore the strengths and weaknesses of proposed strategies is vital to the success of the plan.

Another factor in a successful planning engagement is an absence of critical distractions. Trying to formulate a strategic plan during an employee union drive, in the midst of a financial turnaround, or while the medical staff is waging war on administration is an endeavor destined to fail. If strategic planning is to get the attention it deserves, you must seek a period of time during which major distractions can be minimized.

The quality of the planning engagement can also be improved if you begin preparing for it 6 to 12 months in advance by gathering historical trend information and key performance assessments. Preparing this information in advance will save time when the planning engagement formally begins. It will save money too, since preparing data in-house on history and trends is certain to be cheaper than asking the consulting firm to do it once the planning process has begun.

Creating a sense of positive excitement about the strategic planning process is another factor that can enhance the success of the engagement. When both internal and external constituencies are inspired to focus their creative efforts on planning for the future, the reward is an improved planning engagement. It takes time to identify appropriate external constituencies and to get them excited about participating in the planning process. Regardless of the strategic planning approach, introducing the consultants positively to the organization at the beginning of the engagement is the first step in getting the best work from them.

GETTING THE BEST CONTRIBUTION FROM CONSULTANTS

Preparing strategic planning consultants to work effectively is an important factor in the quality of their contribution to your organization. Time invested in orienting consultants before the beginning of the consultation is one of the best ways to ensure that the consultants are effective.

How should consultants be oriented? First, the consultants need to spend time getting to know the organization's leaders.

Interviews with board, administration, and medical staff leaders present an excellent opportunity for consultants to become familiar with the organization. It is very helpful for the consultants to meet, in an informal setting, at least a dozen of the organization's key leaders before formally beginning the planning engagement. These leaders will eventually form the nucleus of the various planning committees; hearing their perspectives on the past and their hopes for the future of the organization is invaluable. These informal meetings also present the opportunity for the organization's leaders to get to know the consultants, promoting a sense of trust and respect from the start.

Consultants should also get to know a sampling of the organization's employees, middle management staff, and professional/clinical staff. Focus groups can be arranged to give the consultants an opportunity to meet the staff who are the backbone of the organization, the middle managers who oversee the day-to-day work of the organization and the clinical staff who orchestrate the care of patients. Meeting representatives of these three important groups can give the consultants an appreciation of what the organization is really like at the employee, manager, and clinical-staff level. Often the perspective from this level can be quite different from that of senior management, the board, or clinical staff leaders.

Finally, it is very helpful to arrange for the consultants to meet one or two focus groups of current or former patients. This can ground the consultants on perspectives of the customers, a viewpoint that may be different from that of staff or leadership.

While all these introductory meetings and interviews are taking place, the consultants should be given a tour of all of the organization's facilities. The next step in ensuring success is for the chief executive officer to "charge" the consultants to put forth their very best creative effort and to assure them that the organization will encourage and seek out creative discussion. The chief executive should say, in effect, "Don't be afraid to be provocative. Challenge us to think creatively and not be held hostage to the past. Don't let us settle for anything less than achieving our full creative potential." So charged, effective consultants can help clients voice their most precious hopes and creative ideas for the future.

As always, showing respect and commitment for the consultants and their approach to strategic planning will go a long way toward ensuring success for the engagement. Once begun, everyone in the organization should be fully committed to the planning process established by the consultants and focus their energies on avoiding the pitfalls that can cause strategic planning to go awry.

AVOIDING STRATEGIC PLANNING PITFALLS

Disappointments in the strategic planning process can occur during and after the engagement is completed. During the engagement, care should be taken not to completely delegate the creative element of strategic planning to consultants, even if the authored planning approach is used. It is the responsibility of the organization's leadership to articulate a vision of the future and milestones in achieving that vision. Consultants should not be charged with creating a vision for the organization.

Another complication that can derail an effective strategic planning engagement is focus, even obsession, on a particular strategy. It is not uncommon for a chief executive, board member, or clinical staff leader to have a single-minded viewpoint on how to plan for the future. If the planning process is overpowered by a singular viewpoint, the opportunity for creativity is lost.

The opposite situation occurs when a planning engagement unearths so many ideas for the future that they cannot be effectively prioritized or selected for implementation. Having too many good ideas is just as bad as having only one idea. Consultants can help achieve balance in articulating numerous good ideas, but you must have the discipline to choose those that will form the basis of future strategic plans.

Not taking enough time to process ideas and strategies during the engagement is another pitfall. An excellent strategic plan will never emerge from one or two good planning meetings. It emerges through many meetings and drafts and stands the test of debates and thorough discussion. If more time is spent gathering data and researching the past than discussing alternative plans for the future, the quality of the plan is not likely to be good.

A final pitfall to avoid during and after the engagement is assuming the weight or length of the planning document is a measure of quality. There are countless long strategic plans with hundreds of tables of data that gather dust, forgotten on boardroom shelves. Quality is more important than quantity in strategic planning.

While consultants have considerable influence on the quality of the plan during its preparation, the ultimate determining factor of any strategic plan's success rests with the client. Only a successfully implemented plan is worth more than the paper it is printed on. A successful strategic planning engagement is judged by the results the organization achieves based on the plan, not by the plan document. The biggest pitfall of all can be avoided by fully implementing the recommended strategies. Not even the most brilliantly conceived strategic plan can guarantee it will be effectively executed.

Strategic Planning Revolving Door: A community hospital commissioned four strategic plans during a ten-year period. Although the plans were each intended to cover a five-year period, each was abandoned after two years and another strategic plan was started. Four different consulting firms were used to produce these strategic plans, and each firm was abandoned along with their plan after completion.

While the content of the four plans differed, there was a common theme in the strategies. Each plan called for confronting clinical quality problems with powerful members of the medical staff. The first two plans were abandoned after the chief executives were fired attempting to address the quality problems. The second two plans were abandoned when the incumbent chief executive determined his firing would be inevitable if he confronted the powerful physicians in question.

In this case, the fifth attempt succeeded in producing not only a sound strategic plan but also a board and chief executive willing to execute it. The physicians with quality problems were finally confronted and ultimately left the community. They were promptly replaced with better physicians, and the hospital improved both its quality of care and its reputation in the community.

CHECKLIST FOR A SUCCESSFUL PLANNING EXPERIENCE

Strategic planning is an integral part of every successful healthcare enterprise. It can be the catalyst for bringing the organization together and creating a successful future. Strategic planning is an endeavor that absolutely benefits from the involvement of an effective consultant. Steps for a successful experience include the following:

1. *Research.* Review history, trends, and performance before starting the planning process.
2. *Decide.* Decide whether an authored plan or a facilitated plan is better.
3. *Choose.* Hire the very best consultant or consulting firm to help maximize the organization's creative potential.
4. *Allocate.* Set aside enough time and involve enough people to take full advantage of the creative potential of all constituencies.
5. *Discuss.* Debate, refine, and coalesce the full scope of ideas until the best strategies are formulated and prioritized.
6. *Create.* Build consensus around the best strategies.
7. *Implement.* Implement the best strategies and achieve successful outcomes.

CONCLUSION

Successful implementation of recommended strategies is the true measure of success for a strategic plan. Consultants can help organizations map their route to the future, but the organizations themselves must drive the bus to get there. The synergy between capable strategic planning consultants and action-oriented organization leaders makes all the difference between arriving at the desired destination and getting lost or wrecked along the way.

CHAPTER ELEVEN

Legal Consultation

E VERY HEALTHCARE ORGANIZATION uses legal consultants. Many organizations use the same legal advisor or law firm year after year with little or no evaluation of the quality and value of legal services. Healthcare governing boards and chief executives typically do not exercise sufficient due diligence in selecting legal advisors or in periodically evaluating them once they are selected. Governing boards and chief executives need to be much more attentive to the selection and retention of legal consultants. Poor legal advice has contributed to the closure of healthcare organizations. Excellent legal advice can help save an organization from financial and quality problems. In today's environment of heavy corporate compliance and focus on quality, good legal advice can make the difference between thriving as an organization and closing in disgrace.

Healthcare organizations need both general and specialized services from their legal consultants. General counsel services are necessary in even the smallest organizations. The organization's general counsel, either an individual or a law firm, provides overall guidance on legal matters. General counsels are like internal medicine physicians who have broad knowledge about caring for patients and can treat a wide variety of ills but refer their patients to subspecialists when specialized care is needed. General counsels handle the day-to-day routine legal work for their clients but refer them to legal specialists when specific expertise is needed. When the specialty services are no longer necessary, the organization returns to the general counsel for continuing guidance and advice.

This chapter will focus primarily on selecting and getting the best consultation value from general counsel legal consultants.

All long-term consultants, including legal consultants, should be periodically evaluated. Quality of services, quality of communication, and cost/benefit of legal services should be evaluated annually. The chief executive officer, on behalf of the governing board, is best equipped to perform this evaluation. In the absence of evaluation, legal consultants can become "institutionalized." General counsels especially tend to become permanent fixtures of the organizations they advise. It is not uncommon for general counsels to become de facto board members, ever-present at board and important governance committee meetings. The only differences between these de facto board members and elected board members are that general counsels are not subject to term limits and are paid for their presence.

Another potential drawback of the relationship between the board and its legal consultants is that a dependency can be created whereby the board and senior management never contemplate a decision or strategy initiative without first consulting with their general counsel. While this is quite appropriate in some instances it is often a complete waste of time and money. Attorneys are trained to protect their clients' best interests in the event of a worst-case scenario. However, if every organization initiative and strategy undergoes a worst-case scenario analysis, there would be precious little initiative in the healthcare industry.

Legal advisors are vital consultants for all healthcare organizations. But organization leaders must keep in mind that attorneys are consultants. They should never be permitted or encouraged to preempt the judgment of the chief executive or members of the board.

CHOICES AVAILABLE FOR LEGAL SERVICES

Healthcare organizations have many options to choose from when selecting legal consultants, especially general counsels. It is very important that the organization have one attorney or one firm to act as general counsel. The general counsel may be an in-house attorney employed by the organization, or the general counsel may be an independent attorney retained by the organization for that specific role. A law firm retained by the organization can handle the general counsel function even if no specific individual in the firm is designated general counsel to the organization.

However, whenever possible, it is preferable to have a qualified individual serve in this role rather than a law firm.

Healthcare organizations may choose their general counsels from small general law firms, specialty law firms with expertise in healthcare, mid-sized regional law firms with healthcare groups, or large law firms with healthcare departments. Each of these options has unique advantages and disadvantages. Small firms may be in a position to offer more personal service to their clients, but may lack the scope of expertise available in specialty, regional, and large law firms. Regional law firms often have a wide range of expertise available, but may offer less personalized service. Large firms have the widest range of expertise, but often their healthcare practices are secondary to other corporate legal work. Large firms may also have significantly higher fees than small or regional firms.

DEFINING THE OPTIMAL SCOPE OF LEGAL SERVICES

What legal consultation services do general counsels provide? The general counsel plays a very significant role as a trusted advisor to the board and chief executive, helping to determine when specialized legal expertise is needed and where to find the best specialized legal advice. General counsels can also play a very important role in either inflating or deflating the total legal expenses incurred by an organization. Employed (in-house) general counsels tend to increase the overall legal service costs. While this may seem counterintuitive, keep in mind that employed general counsels are in a position to identify more legal work than would be the case if counsel were not in-house. Even the most insignificant contracts and purchase agreements may receive attention by an in-house general counsel eager to prove his or her worth to the organization. If these contracts are specialized in nature, the in-house general counsel may send them to outside legal experts, adding more to the organization's legal expenses. Organizations without in-house counsel may not subject every agreement to legal scrutiny, depending instead on the good judgment of senior management to approve all but the most complicated agreements.

Bogus Deal: A community hospital had used the same local law firm for thirty years. The firm had four partners, one of whom served as the general counsel to the hospital. The general counsel had attended all board meetings for the past 15 years, acting as a member of the board without having been appointed. The attorney approached the board chairman and several other influential board members with a proposal that he join the hospital staff as an in-house general counsel. He emphasized that this strategy would save legal fees "in the long run." The board approved the proposal without consulting with the chief executive officer. This was not a match made in heaven.

As an in-house general counsel, the attorney immediately became a senior vice president on the hospital's administrative staff, causing resentment among the other senior executives. He was the highest paid senior executive, even though he had the least healthcare experience. Before long, the general counsel had inserted himself into virtually every area of the organization, demanding that every management decision have a legal review. An interesting aspect of the increased legal reviews was that the general counsel did not perform these himself. Instead, he referred them to his old law firm and other specialty legal firms. After two years of this arrangement, the hospital's legal expenses had tripled. Twice as many outside law firms were receiving referral business from the general counsel, the hospital was now saddled with its in-house attorney's high salary, and his old law firm was receiving the same amount of legal work from the hospital as it had before the employment arrangement.

To add insult to injury, the in-house general counsel began acting more and more like a board member. He supplied "back channel" commentary to the board on the chief executive and senior management staff that was highly critical. He worked behind the scenes tirelessly to get the chief executive fired and positioned himself to succeed him. Unfortunately for all concerned, the hospital experienced extreme financial distress and nearly declared bankruptcy. A turnaround management team was hired to save the hospital and immediately moved to terminate the general counsel's employment. Since the general counsel had written his own employment agreement, it contained a highly unusual and generous severance package. The general counsel was fired, but he left the hospital a wealthy man.

While a good general counsel can advise on a wide variety of legal matters, it is inevitable that specialized legal services may occasionally be needed, even by the smallest healthcare organizations. Some specialized legal services often utilized by healthcare organizations include corporate compliance, regulatory, tax, clinical/professional staff, risk management, quality of care, malpractice, reimbursement, labor and employment, corporate transactions, contracts, and anti-trust. The list could be endless, depending on the complexity of the organization and the scope of its initiatives.

The environment in which healthcare organizations operate is extremely complicated. Excellent legal consultants are needed to assist organizations in navigating these complex waters and avoiding the many challenges that await the organization. The key to knowing when and who to use as a specialty legal consultant is retaining a very competent and trusted general counsel.

How does the organization go about selecting a good general counsel? Just like any other important consultant selection: very carefully and with a thorough evaluation process.

SELECTING THE BEST LEGAL CONSULTANT

In some healthcare organizations, an appointment as general counsel is the closest thing to a lifetime Supreme Court assignment. Once selected, only retirement or premature death ends the consulting relationship. General counsels often serve far longer than the board members and chief executives who retain them. However, like any other important consultant to the organization, legal advisors should be carefully selected, evaluated annually, and periodically subjected to the request for proposal process to ensure that the best quality and best value of legal advice is received.

> **Time for a Change:** A large urban hospital had used the services of a board member's law firm for several years. All of the organization's legal business filtered through the board member's firm, although he was not personally involved in the hospital's legal business. The amount of legal fees flowing to the firm exceeded half a million dollars a year.
>
> When the board decided to enforce its conflict of interest policy, the board member resigned but requested that his firm retain the hospital's legal business. Instead the board asked the chief executive officer to conduct an RFP selection process. Ten well-qualified firms of all sizes were contacted. This was the first RFP several of the law firms had ever received. The former board member's firm did not receive an RFP because

it was determined that his firm did not have sufficient healthcare expertise to be considered.

After evaluation and personal interviews, the chief executive, with input from the board, chose a new firm to provide general counsel services. Within a year, the new general counsel had favorably resolved several large pending litigations. In addition, legal fees were cut approximately 30 percent because the new firm's billing rates were considerably lower than those of the firm it replaced.

Perhaps most significantly, the new general counsel performed his duties as a true consultant to the board and chief executive. Since the previous firm had one of its senior partners on the board, a true consulting relationship had never developed. Changing law firms for general counsel services saved considerable money while at the same time significantly improving the quality of legal consultation services.

Healthcare organizations should begin with selecting a general counsel, even though specialty legal consultants will be needed from time to time. The general counsel will be a trusted advisor to the governing board, chief executive, and senior management and should be an individual, not a law firm. The critical importance of this decision justifies the time and effort required to use the RFP process.

There are several important criteria on which an RFP can be constructed for legal services. Criteria of particular importance include the following:

1. *Experience.* Experience and expertise in healthcare law is critical. A good track record of serving as a healthcare general counsel is also essential.
2. *Access.* The general counsel must be readily available for questions and crisis management. The organization must be able to reach its general counsel on a moment's notice.
3. *Honesty and integrity.* To be an effective general counsel, the attorney must have impeccable integrity and the ability to deliver honest advice, regardless of the circumstances.
4. *Consulting expertise.* In addition to technical expertise, a good legal advisor will be a good consultant, able to listen effectively, articulate options, and offer sound advice regarding a course of action.

5. *Absence of conflict.* Many opportunities exist for conflicts of interest when using legal consultants. The organization should select a legal advisor with absolutely no potential for conflict of interest.

6. *Impartiality.* A good legal consultant will have the knowledge and skill to assist the organization in selecting the best specialized legal expertise when needed. He or she will also have the integrity to go outside of his or her own law firm for this expertise if it is in the organization's best interest.

7. *Value.* The best general counsel embodies all of the above characteristics plus the ability to use financial resources in a manner that achieves the best legal advice at the lowest cost to the organization.

Healthcare organizations seldom construct an RFP with the above criteria, but it should be routine. A sample RFP for general counsel legal services is provided in Appendix F at the end of this book. Even if the organization's leaders are satisfied with their current legal consultants, they should pursue the legal RFP process every three to five years to ensure they are getting the best legal service at the best possible price. When choosing firms for the RFP process, preliminary research should be performed to determine which law firms are qualified and do not have conflicts of interest. Local hospital associations and bar associations are a good place to begin identifying qualified firms and individuals. Approximately five to ten RFPs can be released to qualified firms and the responses evaluated by the chief executive and board. At least three firms should receive personal interviews and the most qualified and capable general counsel be selected and retained. The consulting arrangement should be evaluated on an annual basis by the chief executive, with the results of the evaluation reported to the governing board.

BOARD AND CHIEF EXECUTIVE OFFICER RESPONSIBILITIES

The governing board and chief executive share responsibility for the organization's legal matters. The board is responsible for overall compliance with the organization's bylaws. In hospitals, the board is also clearly responsible for the appointment and reappointment process for physicians and the quality of care provided by them. The chief executive officer is responsible for hiring and firing the organization's staff and for contractual relationships with service providers. The chief executive is also responsible for financial operations and for numerous contracts and legal agreements. The board and chief executive are jointly responsible for the umbrella of corporate compliance and ensuring that the organization is operated within the nearly infinite regulations and other requirements of local, state, and federal government and accreditation agencies.

Given the critical nature of legal issues confronting healthcare organizations, it is interesting to note that rarely are annual legal reports delivered to governing boards. Boards receive annual financial reports, safety committee reports, human resources reports, and volunteer reports, but seldom receive a legal report covering the year's most important events and expected legal challenges on the horizon for the next year. This is an important communication opportunity that should not be overlooked. At a minimum, the board's annual legal report should include the following:

- The organization's compliance with applicable regulatory requirements
- Status of pending legal actions against the organization
- Status of pending legal actions on behalf of the organization against other organizations
- Anticipated problems or opportunities of a legal nature expected in the coming year
- Summary of all legal costs incurred by the organization during the year compared with previous years' expenses

PITFALLS TO AVOID WITH LEGAL CONSULTANTS

Attorneys, especially general counsels, are very important members of any healthcare organization's consulting team. They perform both episodic project work and long-term advisory services. The governing board and chief executive both benefit from their advice and counsel. As with any consulting engagement, there are several pitfalls that must be avoided. Attorneys should never be permitted to become de facto board members. This sometimes happens when the general counsel becomes a permanent fixture in the organization. There is no reason for this to occur, and no reason why a legal representative should be present at every board meeting. Attorneys are consultants, not decision makers.

Attorneys should not be asked or permitted to evaluate the chief executive or senior management. Because of their status as trusted advisors, they are sometimes asked by board members to provide input on executive evaluations. This is not appropriate, and the practice should be discouraged. In addition, legal advisors should not be part of strategy formation for the organization unless their legal expertise is needed. Attorneys are sometimes asked for input into matters that are beyond their expertise. Boards or chief executives should not look to their legal advisors for financial, strategic, or operational advice.

The practice of employing general counsels should be avoided in all but the largest healthcare organizations with the most complex of legal needs. Employment of in-house general counsels generally does not reduce legal expenses and may restrict the creative and entrepreneurial initiatives undertaken by the organization.

Finally, legal consultants, like all other consultants, should be subject to periodic reviews and evaluations of their performance and value to the organization. No consultant, including an attorney, should be permanently retained by the organization without periodic performance reviews.

CHECKLIST FOR ACHIEVING SUCCESSFUL LEGAL CONSULTATION

The key to obtaining the best possible legal advice is selecting a good general counsel and working closely with him or her to determine when specialized legal advice is needed and who can provide that specialized advice with the highest quality and greatest value. Suggestions for a successful experience with legal consultants include the following.

1. *Review.* Evaluate general counsel legal services annually, using these key criteria:
   - Quality and integrity
   - Availability and access
   - Cost effectiveness
   - Communication skills
   - Advice to board and chief executive officer

2. *Evaluate.* The board and chief executive should use an RFP process every three to five years to select or confirm a general counsel and to ensure that the organization is receiving the highest quality legal advice at the most economical cost.

3. *Communicate.* The organization's legal counsel should provide an annual report to the governing board that highlights the past year's notable legal events as well as prepares the board for the coming year's challenges. A legal audit is just as important as the financial audit that has become a standard annual report to management and the board.

CONCLUSION

Legal consultants, like auditors, are in the unique position of being retained on an ongoing basis by healthcare organizations. The quality of legal advice can make a definitive difference between making consistently sound legal decisions and constantly defending poor legal decisions. The governing board and senior management must make sure they retain the best and most effective general counsel. Careful avoidance of conflicts of interest and routinely evaluating the quality of legal services are the keys to success in working with these important consultants.

Part Three, "Consultants to Management," continues the detailed discussion of how to work most effectively with consultants who are primarily retained by healthcare organization senior management.

PART THREE

Consultants to Management

CHAPTER TWELVE

Improving Financial Performance

FINANCIAL PERFORMANCE IMPROVEMENT is crucial for every healthcare organization. Strong financial performance is the long-term key to success because it ensures that sufficient resources are available to continually update the facility and equipment as well as attracting and retaining the best possible staff and clinicians. When financial performance deteriorates, so does the overall quality of the organization.

A healthcare chief executive can spend a fortune on consulting fees trying to improve financial performance and still get fired. Perhaps there is a cause and effect relationship between spending a virtual fortune and having little or nothing to show for it. Improving financial performance does represent a great opportunity for a chief executive to invest wisely in consulting services and have extraordinarily positive results to show for it. The difference between success and unemployment is knowing when to retain a consultant and how to select the best consulting approach to meet the organization's needs.

Consulting for financial performance improvement offers many benefits. It may, for example, enable an organization with mediocre finances to improve its performance so that it has access to debt markets for adding new facilities or implementing new clinical services. It may enable an organization to provide its services more competitively—an advantage itself in a competitive managed care market. Improved financial performance may give the organization the wherewithal to pay better wages and provide better fringe benefits, enabling it to attract and retain better staff.

Alternatively, attempting to improve financial performance carries big risks. Consulting fees for financial performance improvement can be astronomical. If the organization does not achieve the desired results, it may waste hundreds of thousands of dollars. Poorly executed consultations have been known to disrupt entire delivery systems, alienating both staff and physicians, not to mention patients. Failed financial performance improvement consultations have led to dramatic increases in employee and management turnover.

Financial performance improvement is fraught with risk and rewards. Chief executives must envision the rewards and have the discipline and competence to manage the risks of hiring a financial performance improvement consultant. One certainty is that a chief executive who delays his decision to retain a financial improvement consultant is at a higher risk of being displaced by a turnaround consultant.

WHEN TO RETAIN A PERFORMANCE IMPROVEMENT CONSULTANT

Many healthcare organization leaders wait far too long before arresting a downward trend in financial performance. They often employ half measures and ineffective strategies in the hope that more drastic measures will not be necessary. Unfortunately, this delay often makes the drastic action they seek to avoid inevitable.

When a financially stable healthcare organization has a catastrophic financial loss (5 percent or greater), immediate action must be taken by the organization's leaders to avoid a repeat performance. An organization that experiences two or more years of modest financial losses (1 percent to 3 percent) should also take action to reverse the financial trend. Modest losses tend to become larger and permanent unless intervention is successfully undertaken. A first-time catastrophic loss can spell disaster if it is repeated the following year. Financial losses should not be allowed to continue, period.

Financial performance improvement may also be contemplated for strategic reasons. If the organization needs access to new capital in the form of bond issue debt, improving the bottom line is one essential strategy. Building new facilities or renovating old ones often calls for more capital than can be accumulated through normal operations. Profitable operations enable the organization to borrow responsibly. The more profitable the organization, the better the borrowing rates available to it.

Another strategic reason to improve financial performance is to add value to an organization so its leaders can purchase new enterprises or merge into a larger organization. Improving financial performance can be the key to positioning a strong organization for an acquisition or positioning a weaker organization to achieve its best value in the event it is acquired.

Competitor Beware: The chief executive of the smallest hospital in a three-hospital town conducted a financial performance consultation with an interesting challenge. He proposed doubling his organization's operating margin from 2 percent to 4 percent so he could position his organization to acquire the largest hospital in town. His largest competitor was in its fifth year of significant financial losses.

The chief executive's management staff and physician leaders, in conjunction with the financial performance consultant, examined every conceivable revenue enhancement and cost reduction opportunity and created a list of positive initiatives that added $7 million to the hospital's bottom line.

Without hesitation, all of the initiatives were implemented and the hospital doubled its operating margin to 4 percent as planned. Two years later the hospital initiated a successful merger with its largest competitor. After integrating operations of the two facilities, the new hospital system became the largest provider in the county and one of the most profitable in the state.

It is sometimes difficult to make the decision to engage a financial improvement consultant. Organization leaders may ask themselves the following questions to put the decision into perspective.

- Is operating profitability less than 1 percent?
- Has profitability fallen for more than one year?
- Is financial performance below board expectations?
- Is there a strategic opportunity to expand services in the community?
- Is our credit rating below the "A" level?

If the answer to any of these questions is yes, financial performance must be significantly improved. Once the decision is made to seriously address financial performance improvement, the next challenge is deciding which of the many approaches will lead to success.

ALTERNATIVE APPROACHES TO FINANCIAL PERFORMANCE IMPROVEMENT

Four major approaches are available to improve financial performance. One approach requires no consulting assistance; the other three require consulting assistance ranging from facilitation to large teams of consultants spending months or years working with the organization's leadership. The alternative approaches are discussed below.

Internal Approach

The internal approach to financial performance improvement requires no consulting intervention. If an organization's leaders recognize a need to improve financial performance, they can and should do everything possible to increase revenues and reduce costs to improve the bottom line. This approach is typically used when preparing the organization's annual budget. If the budget for the coming year projects insufficient financial performance, leaders should call for improvement.

While requiring no consulting intervention, the internal approach does require considerable time and commitment. It is customary for the chief executive or chief financial officer to establish a financial improvement target and charge senior management or senior and middle management staff members to achieve the target by either increasing revenue or decreasing costs. Properly motivated management staff can be creative and offer ideas for performance improvement. However, this approach is seldom successful in achieving significant long-term performance improvements because individual managers often feel they are already running their areas of responsibility in the most efficient manner possible. In the absence of an informed opinion to the contrary, they will resist pressure to reduce costs. Unless demands are made for across-the-board cuts, which are highly ineffective, managers are unlikely to make meaningful and sustained changes in their operations. Most will claim that other departments, not theirs, are inefficient and in need of streamlining.

Although not always effective, an internal financial improvement approach should be implemented at least once before proceeding with financial performance approaches that require consulting intervention.

Targeted Approach

The targeted performance improvement approach enables the organization to focus on revenue enhancement or cost reduction in a narrow area without involving the entire organization. Specialty consulting firms are available to assist organizations with the targeted approach. If revenue enhancement is the objective, consultants may be retained to maximize reimbursement, minimize revenue deductions, or use pricing methodologies that increase demand for services. If cost reduction is the objective, consulting firms can help organizations reduce staffing costs, purchase supplies and services more economically, and evaluate programs for potential efficiencies.

The targeted approach usually yields positive results for the organization. There is little organization-wide disruption, and consulting fees are low or moderate. If an organization's leaders know in advance that the targeted approach is likely to yield sufficient financial performance improvement, it is reasonable to pursue this approach before a more comprehensive approach is considered.

Facilitated Approach

The facilitated financial performance improvement approach entails using a consultant to help implement a process of revenue enhancement and cost-reduction initiatives throughout the organization. This approach follows the 80/20 rule: 80 percent of the initiatives originate within the organization and 20 percent originate with the consultant.

In this approach the consultant assists organization leaders to implement a process to stimulate creative ideas to increase revenue and reduce costs. The consultant brings structure and discipline to the process along with experience from other successful performance improvement engagements. The responsibility for initiating the ideas remains with the organization's employees, managers, and clinical staff.

If the consultant is experienced, this approach can be very effective. Because idea generation remains with internal leaders, ownership and implementation can be very effective. This approach assumes that the organization's internal leaders can judge which costs can be reduced without compromising quality and which sources of revenue have the highest potential for increase.

The facilitated approach depends heavily on commitment from the organization's leadership and the availability of sufficient time for the organization's staff to participate fully. Professional fees are low to moderate, and organization disruption is minimal due to the low-key presence of consultants.

Comprehensive Consulting Approach

The comprehensive consulting approach to financial performance improvement could also be labeled the "most" approach. It costs the most money, takes the most time, uses the most consultants, and entails the most organizational disruption.

The comprehensive approach to performance improvement requires the least participation by senior management. In fact, this approach delegates the responsibility for generating revenue enhancement and cost reduction ideas to a team of consultants. Often a dozen or more consultants are required, and it is not uncommon for a comprehensive performance improvement project to take 6 to 12 months. Fees are typically in the seven-figure range. Other than turnaround consultants, comprehensive financial performance improvement consultants are the most expensive consultants a healthcare organization can retain.

To make this approach feasible, the organization's chief executive must be convinced that he or she does not have the time or experience to achieve satisfactory results without a team of consultants. This approach substitutes the organization's money for the organization's time. Less time equals more money in professional fees.

Unfortunately, many healthcare organization leaders jump first to the comprehensive consulting approach. It would be far better to begin with the internal approach and then move to the targeted or facilitated approach if necessary. The comprehensive approach should be considered only as a last resort.

SELECTING THE BEST CONSULTANT

Regardless of which consulting approach is contemplated, the selection of the right consultant is critical to achieving desired results. The targeted, facilitated, and comprehensive approaches for financial performance improvement each have unique consulting perspectives. After selecting the approach which best meets the organization's needs, you must select the best consultant or consulting firm.

The range of options for the targeted approach is limited. Specialty consulting firms or divisions of large firms are options. Technical expertise is the principal consideration in selecting a targeted approach consultant. If the challenge is to increase reimbursement, employee productivity, or supply purchasing effectiveness, a limited number of consulting firms have expertise in this area. When evaluating these firms, three additional criteria are important:

1. Track record of implemented recommendations
2. Sustained results
3. Staff buy-in

Successful targeted approach firms have a client track record of suggestions that were fully implemented with sustained results and staff acceptance of those recommendations.

In the facilitated approach, an ability to work with internal staff to stimulate ideas for performance improvement is the most important skill needed. When evaluating these firms, track record, sustained results, and staff buy-in are also important.

For the comprehensive approach, the leadership, scope, and depth of the consulting team are the principal criteria for evaluating different firms. Typically, the comprehensive approach is only available from large consulting firms or firms that specialize in financial performance improvement. Several turnaround firms also offer this service to financially stable organizations.

As with other types of consulting services, identifying three to five qualified firms and using a request for proposal process is advisable. RFP responses should be evaluated in these key areas:

- The firm's experience in performance improvement
- Assigned consultant's experience
- Methodology
- Professional fees and timeframe
- Professional references

In financial performance improvement consulting, it is extremely important to retain consultants who are compatible with the organization's culture. The last thing you need is a consultant or firm who makes themselves look good at the your expense. Personal interviews and thorough reference checks are essential in selecting the best financial performance improvement consultant. Once the selection is made, you should prepare to achieve the full value of the consultation.

PREREQUISITES FOR A SUCCESSFUL OUTCOME

The most decisive factor in achieving success in a financial performance improvement engagement is neither the approach nor the consultant. It is the commitment of the organization's management, specifically its chief executive officer. If you need or want to improve your organization's financial performance, you cannot succeed by delegating this assignment to a consultant. The right consultant *can* be an enormous help, but it is the organization itself that controls whether the endeavor is a success or a failure.

What do you need to do to ensure success? First, there should be a clear purpose and a definitive goal for financial performance improvement. Making a bigger profit or cutting a loss is too nebulous an objective. The goals should be supported by an important achievement for the organization. Good examples are, "We need to improve profit margins from 1 percent to 2 percent to achieve a sufficiently favorable bond rating to replace our outdated surgery suite," or "We need to reduce our operating loss from $5 million to less than $1 million to have sufficient cash reserves to weather a Medicare reimbursement slowdown." In other words, create a goal that all staff can understand and support.

Second, the organization's entire leadership must support the financial performance improvement goal. The chief executive must be willing and able to rally his or her troops around the goal. Each member of senior management and the clinical staff leadership must support the goal if the project is to succeed. Some leaders believe hiring consultants is a substitute for personal commitment. Nothing could be further from the truth. Without leadership's personal commitment, millions can be spent on financial performance improvement consultants without achieving any results.

Another important factor for success is the ability of the organization's leadership to put politics and "sacred cows" aside. It is difficult, if not impossible, to motivate employees and managers to seek ways to cut costs if favored clinical staff or executives receive special perks or considerations. Take away the sacred cows, and organizations are often rewarded with tremendously creative ideas from their staffs.

Organization leaders need to trust their staffs and middle managers. If a laboratory manager says she can reduce one staff position on the evening shift, her supervising vice president should trust that she can achieve the savings while maintaining quality services. It is ironic that senior managers seem to put more trust in outside consultants than they do in their staff and managers, who own the process that is being examined.

Finally, if you desire to achieve the best results from financial performance improvement engagements, you must be prepared to implement the initiatives that your staff and consultant prepare. Nothing is more discouraging than spending precious time and money for a financial performance improvement consultant only to have senior management fail to follow through and not implement recommended initiatives. If a chief executive is not committed to implement financial improvement initiatives, the next consultant that should be engaged by the organization is an executive search consultant.

An organization's leadership must be fully committed to achieve the desired results. Avoiding certain pitfalls will also help the organization succeed.

PITFALLS TO AVOID IN FINANCIAL PERFORMANCE IMPROVEMENT

The biggest pitfall to avoid in financial performance improvement is waiting too long to begin the process. Organization leaders have a tremendous capacity to rationalize a grim financial picture. They convince themselves that improvement is just around the corner, when often it is not even on the block. When a healthcare organization is losing money, its leaders need to initiate actions immediately to eliminate financial losses as quickly as possible. Making excuses is a waste of time. Even nonprofit organizations must be profitable. After all, the nonprofit designation is a tax status, not a financial performance goal.

Hiring turnaround consultants to act as financial performance improvement consultants is another pitfall. Often these firms are oriented toward working with highly distressed organizations in which top management has been or is about to be fired. While turnaround consultants may have the technical skills to help an organization improve financial performance, often they do not have the skills to perform their work in a manner that is positively received by the organization's staff. Hiring your audit firm for financial performance improvement advice should also be avoided. Doing so creates a major conflict of interest that makes it nearly impossible for an effective consulting relationship to be developed.

Poor communication is another problem. If the organization's leaders clearly communicate with staff and clinicians the purpose, approach, and goals of a financial performance improvement engagement, they will usually be receptive. If, however, little or no communication is offered, panic often results.

Avoiding the "hard" decisions that often arise during a financial performance improvement engagement is another danger to avoid. It may be unpopular to discontinue a clinical program, reduce a department's hours of operation, or eliminate a management position in the interest of saving money. If the organization's leaders avoid these politically sensitive decisions, they will find themselves with a demoralized staff that is unwilling to make the concessions necessary to make financial performance improvement work throughout the organization.

Finally, one of the worst things an organization's leaders can do in the midst of financial performance improvement engagement is to exempt senior management from any changes. For example, if a major staff reduction is contemplated, then senior management must contemplate reducing its staffing. If the home care staff must give up their hospital-provided cars to save money, so should the vice presidents. Senior executives should set a positive example for the organization. To do less is nothing short of hypocritical.

CHECKLIST FOR SUCCESSFUL FINANCIAL PERFORMANCE IMPROVEMENT

If at all possible, healthcare organization leaders should address financial performance challenges internally. If internal intervention is insufficient, leaders should have the foresight to retain consultants who can help their organization achieve its financial performance goals. Care should be taken in retaining and using consultants, however. Following are six suggestions for a successful experience.

1. *Define the scope.* Use the lowest levels of consulting intervention first. Targeted or facilitated financial performance consultants should always be used before the organization is subjected to the cost and disruption of the comprehensive approach.
2. *Retain the best.* Choosing the best quality consultant is absolutely essential for financial performance improvement. Check references carefully and be prepared to pay high professional fees to the best consultant.
3. *Prepare.* Communicate the goal and purpose of financial performance improvement to the entire organization before the engagement begins. Provide progress reports frequently throughout the engagement to minimize nervousness.
4. *Trust.* Trust the organization's managers and consultants to identify initiatives that will improve financial performance without compromising quality.
5. *Implement.* Follow through and implement financial performance improvement recommendations. Monitor results carefully to ensure desired improvement goals are achieved.
6. *Follow up.* Perform an "audit" six months after implementation to verify that overall financial performance is on target to meet goals. Make adjustments if necessary.

CONCLUSION

Financial performance improvement is an ongoing challenge. It should become part of the organization's culture so that periodic consulting projects are unnecessary. The highest compliment that can be paid to a consultant in this area is when the organization's managers internalize the skills used during the consulting engagement so that return engagements to improve financial performance are unnecessary.

Clinical performance improvement shares many of the same challenges as financial performance improvement. The use of consultants in this area is explored in the next chapter.

CHAPTER THIRTEEN

Improving Clinical Performance

C LINICAL PERFORMANCE IMPROVEMENT should be an on-going priority of every chief executive, every manager, and every physician associated with a healthcare organization. Unfortunately, maintaining the status quo is the more modest goal to which some healthcare organizations aspire. Clinical performance improvement is a hallmark of successful healthcare organizations. The commitment to constantly improve the quality of service for patients is very hard work.

There is no substitute for strong leadership in achieving optimal clinical performance. Senior clinical executives, medical staff officers, and physician department chairs are all instrumental in achieving and maintaining high quality clinical performance. If any one of these leaders is indifferent, problems will follow that can only be addressed by the organization's chief executive. If he or she is indifferent, clinical performance will be mediocre at best. Leadership, not consulting, is the key to successful clinical performance. Consultants can play a supporting role in the pursuit of optimal clinical performance. The objective of this chapter is to determine when consultants can add value and to identify the steps to ensure that a successful consultation supports the organization's quality improvement goals.

The quality of clinical performance is the combined result of three vital components of the healthcare system: systems, technology, and people. When all three components are deployed effectively, healthcare organizations deliver optimum quality of care. When any one of these three components is lacking, quality is compromised. To achieve and sustain excellent clinical performance, constant review and refinement of all three components is required. Although most organizations have internal resources to evaluate their systems, technology, and people, it can be difficult to achieve a truly objective evaluation. In these instances consultants may prove to be useful as organizations strive to improve quality.

Emergency in the Emergency Room: The emergency room of a large urban hospital with a high patient volume (50,000 visits a year) was experiencing long patient waiting time, triple the normal "walk out" rate, low staff morale, and extreme patient dissatisfaction with quality of care according to attending physicians elsewhere in the hospital. The problems were so enormous and multifaceted that the hospital did not know where to begin to fix them.

After seeking input from key medical staff and management leaders, the chief executive decided to retain an outside consulting firm. Consultants from several small firms, one large accounting firm with a medical division, and a large emergency medicine physician contract firm were considered. A small firm led by a former emergency medicine specialist was ultimately retained. With the help of an internal team comprising hospital physicians, management, and nursing leaders, the consultant soon discovered that the critical problem centered on the physicians in the emergency room.

A local physician group provided emergency medicine services in the hospital. The group in turn contracted with moonlighting medical residents to provide coverage. Because the medical residents were inexperienced in emergency medicine, emergency room care became a series of bottlenecks. Residents ordered more diagnostic tests than experienced emergency medical physicians. Laboratory, radiology, and cardiology diagnostic services could not keep up with the demand. Slow treatment of patients led to long waiting times and the high rate of patient walk outs.

The hospital/consultant team recommended replacement of the medical residents with experienced emergency medicine physicians. The local contract physician group refused to comply and was fired. A group of experienced emergency room physicians was soon recruited, and their arrival alleviated nearly all of the clinical performance problems. Not surprisingly, the number of physicians on duty actually decreased, but their quality of care was so high that they were able to process patients much more quickly than the residents they replaced.

WHEN CONSULTANTS ADD VALUE

Consultants add value to a healthcare organization's pursuit of clinical performance improvement in four important ways: experience, facilitation, overcoming barriers, and training. Clinical performance is a function of systems, technology, and people. If an organization's leaders endeavor to improve radiology services, they should study all three components. Consultants can be used selectively, focusing on only one aspect. It is also possible to use a consultant or consulting firm well versed in radiology services to look at all three quality components. A myriad of details affect clinical quality in any given department. To improve the quality of radiology services, organization leaders need to look at the underlying systems, technology, and staffing issues. Scheduling, image processing, professional interpretation, results reporting, and patient communication systems all have relevance in the radiology department.

Technological factors such as the quality and age of the imaging equipment, maintenance status, image clarity, processing time, and calibration also have relevance to the quality of radiology services. People may be the most important factor in determining quality. The training, competence, and communication skills of the radiologist and staff are very important. When systems or technology are lacking, skilled staff can often compensate. However, when the staff is lacking, no level of technology or system efficiency will enable the organization to offer the optimal level of quality clinical services.

Virtually everything that happens in a healthcare organization has a clinical quality component. Several areas of clinical quality lend themselves to ongoing performance improvement. In a hospital setting the following areas are particularly important:

- Hospital-based physician services (including, emergency medicine, radiology, pathology, and anesthesiology)
- Internal medicine services
- Surgical services
- Obstetrics services
- Cardiology services
- Rehabilitation services
- Nursing services
- Utilization management

All of these clinical services have the three components of systems, technology, and people. Healthcare organizations should strive to continuously evaluate, refine, and improve these services to achieve optimum clinical performance. Skilled consultants are available in each of these clinical areas to complement the organization's internal expertise.

DEFINING THE ENGAGEMENT SCOPE

Before defining the scope of a clinical performance consulting engagement, it is appropriate to state that clinical performance improvement lends itself to the use of internal resources. The use of consultants should be avoided unless the expertise is not available internally. Often internal expertise is available in the systems and technology areas, but not necessarily in the people area. Even if expertise is available in the people area, it may be difficult to judge colleagues and coworkers objectively. In that circumstance, outside consultation can be beneficial.

If outside consultation is necessary for any of the three areas, the first challenge is to define the clinical performance issue as a problem or an opportunity. If, for example, the issue is reducing the number of walk outs in the emergency room, the challenge is to solve a quality problem. On the other hand, if the issue is reducing the acute care hospital stay for stroke patients so they can begin rehabilitation sooner, the challenge may be appropriately labeled as an opportunity. In a third instance, no problem or opportunity is immediately discernable. The organization's leaders may wish to audit clinical performance in the obstetrics unit to determine if improvements in systems, technology, or people could lead to better quality of care. While it is true that most consultations involve solving a known problem or developing a known opportunity, healthcare organization leaders would do well to consider an audit of quality to actively seek out problems or opportunities before they become apparent.

After defining the problem or opportunity, the next challenges are identifying internal resources and defining the desired outcome. In the emergency room walk out rate example, appropriate internal resources would be the physician chief of emergency medicine, the emergency room nursing director, staff physicians and nurses, and heads of support services such as laboratory, radiology, and cardiology that interface with the emergency room. Once the internal resource team is assembled, a desired outcome for the consultation should be articulated. For example, reducing the walk out rate from 3 percent to 1 percent would be an appropriate goal.

Barriers to studying and improving the problem or opportunity under consideration should be identified next. For example, are emergency room physicians likely to change their clinical practices to lower the walk out rate? Do they even care about the walk out rate? Can the laboratory and radiology departments speed up emergency room test results, or are they constrained by lack of resources? Barriers to change should be identified to the extent possible before consideration is given to hiring a consultant. Sometimes merely identifying the barriers presents a potential solution to the quality problem.

If the decision is made to proceed with retaining a consultant, the internal team should clearly define the problem, the expected outcome, and barriers to change. These key items, along with a background statement about the organization, comprise the basis of a good request for proposal (RFP) for clinical performance improvement. Once the RFP is developed, the appropriate organization leaders should identify three to five qualified consultants to evaluate. Professional colleagues, hospital and medical associations, and area academic medical centers are all excellent sources of potential consultants. Also, a literature search of current professional publications is likely to identify other consulting candidates specific to the clinical quality issue.

SELECTING THE BEST CONSULTANT

When RFP responses are received, three important factors should be compared to identify the consultants who may be best suited to assist with clinical performance improvement: consulting methodology, reference checks, and personal interviews. The proposed engagement timeframe and professional fees for the engagement are also important.

The consulting methodology—how the consultation will be performed and by whom—is like a window to the consultant's philosophy. Some performance improvement consulting firms use one or two experts as the primary consulting team. These consultants are usually highly qualified in their area of expertise and have the ability to size up problems and opportunities and propose alternatives for consideration. Other consulting firms use a team of people, including both senior and junior consultants. The professionals assigned to the consulting team form the basis of the consulting methodology. The approach most compatible with the organization's needs should be chosen.

For clinical performance consultants to be successful, they must have excellent interpersonal and technical skills. Reference checking should help determine if both skill sets are present. Reference checks on physician consultants should focus on consulting skills in addition to medical background. Success as a practicing physician does not necessarily translate into success as a consultant. Reference checks should also include confirmation that the consultants were able to help other organizations effect and sustain positive change. Writing a good report is not the most desirable skill in a clinical performance consultant; however, the ability to help implement positive change is, and should be verified during reference checks.

After the RFP and reference checking process has narrowed the field to several qualified consultants, personal interviews should follow. The internal team involved with the clinical performance issue should be included in the personal interviews and final selection of the consultant. Personal interviews enable you to choose the consultant or consulting team most compatible with your organization's culture.

Professional fees, although a large consideration, are not the most important factor when selecting finalists for consideration. The very best consultants usually command the highest fees. In the area of clinical performance improvement, it is usually unwise to select the lowest bidder. It is far better to select the most capable consultant and then negotiate a mutually acceptable professional fee. The engagement timeframe is also an important consideration. The consultant selected must be able to complete the engagement on a schedule that meets the organization's needs.

Anesthesia Dilemma: The chief of surgery of an urban medical center grew increasingly concerned about the quality of anesthesia service available at his hospital. He feared that some of the anesthesiologists were "sloppy" due to advanced age. He felt that ongoing quality reviews were highly inadequate. After several untoward mishaps in the operating room, he approached his colleague, the chief of anesthesiology, with his concerns. He was told to "mind his own business."

The chief of surgery next approached the medical center's chief executive and the chief of the medical staff. They jointly agreed that an outside quality review was necessary and again approached the chief of anesthesiology for cooperation. They too were rebuffed. The chief of anesthesiology threatened to "bring in the lawyers" if any further action was taken against his department. They continued despite the threat.

The chief of surgery, chief of the medical staff, and medical center chief executive surveyed the options for consulting assistance and determined that the nearby university teaching hospital and several national consulting firms provided that service. After conducting an RFP process and interviews, the medical center selected the most qualified (and most expensive) anesthesia consulting proposal. A thorough quality audit followed that identified two anesthesiologists who were lacking in clinical skills and were probably medically impaired. The chief of anesthesiology again refused to act. Subsequently, the medical center executed its prerogative to terminate the contract with the anesthesiologists, and a new group was recruited with the enthusiastic support of the medical staff in general and the department of surgery in particular.

The anesthesiology consultants added significant value to this situation by bringing a knowledgeable quality perspective. Their expertise, along with the resolve of the chief of surgery, chief of the medical staff, and medical center chief executive, brought a very sensitive quality problem to a successful conclusion.

PREREQUISITES FOR A SUCCESSFUL ENGAGEMENT

As with other types of consulting engagements, preparation is critical to the ultimate success of a clinical performance improvement engagement. To achieve excellent results, you must be fully cognizant of the problem or opportunity to be addressed and, more importantly, fully committed to give the engagement the best possible chance of succeeding. How is this accomplished?

Assign the best possible internal leaders to work with the consultants. This can be a problem since the best people are likely to be occupied with their day-to-day jobs. However, you must ensure they are available and have the time to devote to the engagement once it begins. It does no good to hire gifted consultants and expect them to succeed without a dedicated internal team to work with.

A second prerequisite for success is making the time to present and discuss alternatives. Rarely do clinical performance improvement challenges respond to one brilliant insight. Rather, the discussion of alternatives and the refinement of ideas is the likely pathway to success.

Consultants and internal leaders should be given sufficient time to fully explore alternatives.

Lastly, as with other consulting engagements, excellent communication before the consultation begins prepares the organization and minimizes the rumors often associated with performance improvement initiatives. Further suggestions for a successful engagement are noted in the checklist at the end of this chapter.

PITFALLS TO AVOID WITH CLINICAL PERFORMANCE IMPROVEMENT

Once the engagement has begun, attention must be given to avoiding pitfalls that could limit the engagement's success. The biggest pitfall in clinical performance improvement is avoidance. Clinical performance should be viewed in the same manner as financial performance. The financial performance of an organization is continually audited, but how often is clinical performance audited? Not often enough in most organizations.

A healthcare organization should routinely schedule clinical performance audits. If such a schedule were in place, far fewer clinical performance problems would exist. Since this is not usually the case, clinical problems or opportunities that arise should be aggressively pursued. What can go wrong during this pursuit?

One pitfall that can deter improving clinical performance is the "sacred cow." If the clinical issue centers on a poorly functioning but popular nurse, the resolve to change or remove the nurse may not be present. If an opportunity to improve performance might negatively affect the practice of a revered physician, again the resolve may not be present. To truly address clinical performance improvement, sacred cows cannot exist.

> **Heart Dilemma:** A community hospital had only one cardiologist on staff. The hospital learned through market research that 80% of community residents needing cardiology services were leaving the community to find them. The hospital chief executive informally surveyed the medical staff leadership and found that local physicians were referring their patients out of town because of quality concerns about the local cardiologist. They qualified their remarks by emphatically stating that they would not "go public" with their concerns about a well-liked colleague.

The chief executive approached the cardiologist with the offer to recruit a partner for his practice. The cardiologist refused, saying he was as busy as he wanted to be and satisfied with his practice. After evaluating several consulting options, the chief executive retained the chief of cardiology at the state university medical center. The consulting cardiologist determined that the community needed three cardiologists to meet local heart care needs.

The hospital, with the support of the university medical center, undertook a successful recruitment for a new cardiologist. After six months, the new cardiologist recruited a partner. The original cardiologist stayed on and prospered. His original concerns proved to be unfounded. Two years later, all three cardiologists enjoyed thriving practices. Follow-up market research showed that half the community residents were receiving their heart care locally. Without the sound advice of a qualified consultant and the firm resolve of the hospital's chief executive, this opportunity for increased quality would have remained unrealized.

Rushing to a solution can derail a clinical performance improvement initiative. If a technology problem is detected early in the review process, it should never preempt a thorough review of the systems and people component of the issue. More than one quality initiative has been prematurely stopped because the answer appeared obvious. Later, the situation proved more complicated than at first glance and the solution not at all obvious.

Another pitfall that can negatively affect clinical improvement initiatives is poor communication. Unless all constituencies understand the problem or opportunity, they may very well resist proposed solutions. Good communication throughout the engagement is very important.

The biggest pitfall of all is failing to implement an identified solution. Clinical performance improvement often involves changing embedded systems, technology, and people. While there is rarely resistance to changing technology, there is almost always resistance to changing systems and people. When a clinical performance improvement consultation reaches its conclusion, sometimes implementation of proposed recommendations requires making system or personnel changes that seem impossible. The organization's leaders may withdraw support for challenging solutions because initiating them might be politically difficult. Unless you are fully committed to quality improvement, the time, energy, and money spent on the consultation is wasted.

CHECKLIST FOR A SUCCESSFUL CLINICAL PERFORMANCE IMPROVEMENT ENGAGEMENT

Clinical performance improvement should be one of the most important priorities of any healthcare organization. In many organizations it achieves this status; in others, blatant neglect is more common. Some suggestions to succeed in clinical performance improvement follow.

1. *Audit.* Routinely audit key clinical services. To be objective, audits should cover the quality aspects of systems, technology, and people. Audit results should routinely lead to performance improvements.
2. *Use internal resources.* Internal leaders are the best source of clinical performance improvement initiatives (unless they themselves are the problem). Before outside consultants are retained, internal leaders should be given the opportunity to conduct performance audits and tackle clinical performance challenges or opportunities.
3. *Define.* Clearly define the clinical performance problem or opportunity before deciding if outside consultation is necessary.
4. *Establish goals.* Clearly articulate the goal to be achieved before undertaking a clinical performance improvement initiative.
5. *Evaluate consultants.* When consultants are necessary, use a request for proposal process to narrow the selection to several excellent choices. Use reference checks and personal interviews to select the best consultant.
6. *Commit.* Absolutely commit to making the necessary changes to improve clinical performance.
7. *Re-audit.* When improvements are implemented to achieve improved clinical performance, re-audit the process in 6 to 12 months to verify that the initiatives worked as planned.

CONCLUSION

Clinical performance improvement is a never-ending process for even the best healthcare organizations. For poor or mediocre healthcare organizations, it can be a never-begun process. Consultants can assist healthcare organizations to ensure that they achieve and sustain excellent clinical performance.

Another area in which healthcare organizations can make a major impact on quality is customer service performance. As discussed in the next chapter, consultants can offer fresh perspectives that support service quality initiatives.

CHAPTER FOURTEEN

Improving Customer Service

ALL HEALTHCARE ORGANIZATIONS should aspire to achieve superb customer service. Many succeed admirably, while others seek shelter with the inadequate adages, "We're no worse than anyone else" and "If it isn't broke, don't fix it." It is doubtful they will print either phrase on their letterhead or use it as a theme for advertising and marketing campaigns. The quality of an organization's customer service emanates from its leadership quality, just as financial and clinical performance do. Good leadership, personally committed to excellent customer service, can achieve great success in this area. If the leadership component is absent, no amount of consulting can create excellent quality customer service.

Customer service is the total experience of all who receive services from a healthcare organization. It is a cumulative experience, including the experience before, during, and after the delivery of healthcare services. For an outpatient radiology patient, customer service includes scheduling the procedure, arriving at the facility, waiting for the service to be performed, undergoing the exam, hearing about the results, and, finally, receiving the bill for services rendered. For a physician office patient, customer service includes scheduling an appointment, waiting in the office, interacting with the staff and physician during the visit, coordinating care with other physicians, following up with any questions, and receiving the bill for services rendered. This broad interpretation of customer service performance places a burden on healthcare organizations to focus on the

165

entire spectrum of customer experiences, not just the moment an x-ray is completed, a lab test is undergone, or a physical is performed.

Why is customer service performance important? Customers of healthcare organizations use service quality as a surrogate measure of clinical quality. Clinical quality may be superb, but if care is delivered by surly nurses in a messy facility, customers may interpret the entire experience negatively and take their business elsewhere. Customers will relate their experiences to family members, friends, and acquaintances. These commentaries will enhance or diminish the healthcare organization's reputation. In addition, customers view service quality as a component of the overall value of services rendered. Excelling in customer service may enable a healthcare organization to be competitive even if it does not possess the latest medical technology or the most beautiful facility.

Customer service performance emanates from the healthcare organization's leadership. The chief executive, senior management, and professional staff leaders set the tone for customer service quality by their personal example. A chief executive who surrounds him- or herself with overtly unfriendly vice presidents is unlikely to establish a customer-friendly culture. As leaders form the organization's corporate culture, they either encourage customer service to flourish or make it impossible for excellent customer service to exist.

In some organizations, leadership commitment to excellent customer service is so strong that consulting assistance is completely unnecessary. In other circumstances, a leadership team may use consultants' skills to enhance the organization's customer service performance. In those unfortunate organizations where leaders are indifferent to customer service performance, even the most gifted consultants cannot make a sustained difference. This chapter will offer insights on how consultants may be useful in developing and maintaining excellent customer service performance.

WHEN A CUSTOMER SERVICE PERFORMANCE CONSULTANT ADDS VALUE

Leading a healthcare organization successfully is an extraordinarily difficult challenge. Successful chief executives must prioritize organization commitments and resources. Both clinical and financial performance quality are of paramount importance. Why be in business unless the organization can deliver a quality clinical service in a financially responsible manner? Many chief executives in the business world value customer service performance as an organization priority. Among these chief executives were a few so powerfully committed—for example, Walt Disney and Sam Walton—that their leadership example alone created a corporate culture that excels at customer service.

Even the best healthcare organizations can fall short of excellence in customer service. They rely on personal commitment to customer service by their chief executives, supplemented by a strong corporate culture, service-oriented systems and employees, and user-friendly facilities. Customer service consultants have a positive role to play even with these organizations. Consultants can help organize, refine, and implement customer service initiatives. While they cannot substitute for good leadership, consultants can enhance leadership's influence.

Customer service performance consultants add value to healthcare organizations in several important ways. First, they can provide objective evaluations of the customer experience. It is difficult, if not impossible, for an organization's management to be completely objective about its services. It is common, even among good managers, to get defensive when informed about lapses in customer service. Consultants can listen objectively to the customers, record both positive and negative experiences, and communicate them impartially to managers without eliciting defensive responses.

Another aspect of objectivity that consultants may bring is evaluating customer contacts. Managers are under constant pressure to keep positions filled within their departments, juggling the needs of staff and the needs of the department. Sometimes managers may "put up" with less-than-optimal employee attitudes or customer service skills in the interest of keeping a position filled. Think of the nurse manager who tolerates a staff nurse with very poor customer service skills because her only option is to replace him with an agency nurse at three times the cost.

Customer service performance consultants also have a wealth of experience with past clients and know which service ideas work well and which fail miserably. Organization leaders who strive to improve customer service performance can avoid costly mistakes by using a consultant's experience. Finally, the best consultants are able to discern an organization's unique strengths and help the organization's leaders turn not only weaknesses, but also strengths, into customer service perform-ance initiatives.

Consultants cannot add value to an organization that does not truly care about or prioritize customer service. As with other kinds of con-sulting, some leadership teams think they can hire a customer service performance consultant to transform them into highly functioning cus-tomer service providers. They are wrong. These organizations would be better off investing in executive search consultants to replace their in-different leaders.

DEFINING THE ENGAGEMENT SCOPE

A comprehensive customer service performance improvement consult-ing engagement includes five components:

1. Customer research
2. SWOT (strengths, weaknesses, opportunities, and threats) analysis
3. Barriers to improvement
4. Initiatives for improvement
5. Action plan and implementation schedule

These five components comprise the basis for a request for proposal (RFP). A brief synopsis of each follows.

- *Customer research.* Consultants, in conjunction with management staff, should conduct on-site research on the experiences of cus-tomers. Research should include, at a minimum, focus groups, personal interviews of current customers, and telephone surveys of former customers.
- *SWOT analysis.* Using the information gathered during the research process, consultants should work with managers and staff to objectively identify the strengths and weaknesses of the customer experience for each of the services under consideration. If there are nearby competitors, the consultants should make an assessment of the competitors' customer service strengths and weaknesses, which can be viewed as both opportunities for and threats to your organization.

- *Barriers to improvement.* Using their professional experience, consultants should articulate the barriers to improving customer service performance. Barriers could include consideration of facility, equipment, systems, and people.
- *Initiatives for improvement.* The combined creativity and experience of the staff, consultants, and customers should be used to identify initiatives to improve the customer service experience. Initiatives should identify the resources necessary for implementation.
- *Action plan and implementation schedule.* Consultants should develop recommendations based on their cumulative experience and professional judgment. Recommendations should include an implementation plan and timetable, as well as a process to monitor success or failure of the recommended initiatives.

These five elements may be used as the scope of the engagement section of an RFP for a customer service performance improvement engagement for either a narrowly defined engagement for a specific service such as outpatient surgery, or a comprehensive engagement such as an entire hospital. After preparing the RFP for distribution, the next step is selecting the best consultant.

SELECTING THE BEST CUSTOMER SERVICE CONSULTANT

Customer service performance improvement consultants are available through specialized consulting firms or large management consulting firms with customer service divisions. The names of such firms are usually available from regional hospital associations, consultant reference services, and professional associations for customer service improvement consultants.

Select three to five qualified firms for RFP releases. Once RFPS have been received, apply four criteria to narrow the list to finalist firms:

1. Experience of consulting team
2. Track record of consulting firm
3. Methodology
4. Professional fees

The most critical factor is the experience of the consultants proposed for the engagement. You should seek consultants who have successfully worked with organizations to make sustained improvements in customer service. The ability to be objective as well as to motivate is very desirable. Although the track record of the consulting firm is important, it is not as important as the consultants assigned to the engagement. Also evaluate the proposed consulting methodology for compatibility with the organization's culture. Of course, professional fees should always be a consideration.

Once the list of potential consultants has been narrowed to several finalists, reference checks and personal client visits should be the next step. Check references for engagements that ended one or two years previously to determine whether the consultant's recommendations had a sustained effect.

Most importantly, personal visits should be made to organizations served by the finalists' firms. There is absolutely no better way to judge the results of a customer service performance improvement engagement than to visit an organization and come away so impressed with the experience that the choice of consultants is obvious. Most consulting firms would be thrilled to "show off" a previous client to a prospective client. Reluctance to do so could mean that the firm was not nearly as successful as their promotional material asserts.

Results of the RFP process followed by reference checks and personal visits should enable you to easily select the best customer service performance consultant. As with other types of consulting, the consultation methodology should mesh well with your organization's culture. Professional fees are also important but should not be the sole basis for consultant selection. Once the selection is finalized, set the stage for a successful outcome.

PREREQUISITES FOR A SUCCESSFUL CONSULTATION

Commitment by the appropriate leader is the most important prerequisite for success in any customer service performance improvement endeavor. The chief executive officer must be visibly supportive of the effort. If a specific department or service is striving to improve, the senior manager in charge of the service or department must be visibly engaged and supportive. In addition to top management support, staff must also value customer service performance and be committed to improvement. If the department manager wants improvement but employees are indifferent or hostile, the desired improvement will never take place. It is leadership's job to put employees in the appropriate frame of mind. Consultants cannot accomplish this task.

Organization leaders who wish to improve customer service must demand a thoroughly objective assessment of current performance. Defensiveness on the part of organization leaders slows down or stops progress. Reward staff and managers for improvements in customer service and punish staff and managers for failure to support customer service performance initiatives. While this may sound cruel, it is a waste of your resources to focus on customer service improvement only to have certain employees or managers ignore the initiatives and continue to do business as usual.

Finally, to be successful you must make customer service performance a permanent part of your organization's culture. Mixed signals or lack of continuing emphasis will only lead to declining performance.

From Cover Story to Unemployment in Four Short Years: A new chief executive of a large community hospital decided to make customer service the cornerstone of his presidency. He was personally committed to making monumental changes in his hospital's service delivery, and he made it clear that he expected no less from his managers and employees.

The hospital retained a well-known customer service improvement consultant. Working at all levels to improve service, a comprehensive plan was developed and implemented over a one-year period. Employees, managers, and senior executives enthusiastically embraced the focus on customer service performance. The program more than met everyone's expectations. One year later, patient satisfaction scores skyrocketed. Two years later, the hospital's chief executive received national recognition for his customer service improvement successes.

Three years later things had changed. The chief executive, worried about declining financial performance, shifted his focus to "reengineering" the hospital. A large consulting firm was retained for a seven-figure consulting fee. Over the next year the reengineering project involved changing job descriptions and systems throughout the hospital in a comprehensive effort to reduce staffing levels. Employees became disillusioned. Physicians grumbled about declines in clinical quality and service. Patient volume plummeted, and financial performance declined to a 10-year low.

Four years after achieving national acclaim for customer service, the chief executive was fired. His successor inherited a thoroughly demoralized organization where employees bitterly accused the former chief executive of being more interested in personal publicity than the welfare of his hospital.

PITFALLS TO AVOID WITH CUSTOMER SERVICE CONSULTATIONS

Absent or insincere support by the chief executive or departmental leader is the biggest pitfall to avoid in a customer service improvement engagement. Another pitfall concerns consultants and their methodology. Some customer service performance consultants have been compared unfavorably with television evangelists. They organize revival-like meetings, encourage singing or cheerleading sessions, and attempt to create cult-like devotion to customer service. While entertaining, this approach to customer service performance improvement is usually short-lived. When the consultant/cult leader leaves the scene, he pulpit is bare and no one is left to lead the revival.

Another pitfall to avoid is to focus exclusively on employees instead of frontline managers. Several years ago, "guest relations" was a frequently used methodology for customer service performance improvement. This approach concentrated on training employees to be friendlier and more service oriented. While ideal, often this approach failed to reach the middle managers supervising frontline employees. If managers are not on board, training employees to smile does not last long.

As with clinical quality performance, "sacred cows" can be a major hazard for customer service performance improvement. If an employee, a department or service, or a physician is exempted from service quality standards, the entire organization's effort to improve may be compromised.

Finally, inflexible management, at any level, can be a major pitfall of customer service performance improvement initiatives. If management does not trust staff to make good judgments and exceptions to established policies, customer service will never thrive.

Humbling Lesson: A new chief executive in a community hospital was devoted to making customer service performance a large part of the organization's competitive strategy. While it was the smallest hospital in its market, he reasoned it could be the best at customer service, ensuring enough market share to survive.

After two years of strong focus on service quality, he believed his organization was making excellent progress. That is, until the morning he heard a story about two intensive care nurses on the previous night shift. An elderly patient was dying of cancer but still alert and able to enjoy visitors. That evening he requested permission for his nine-year-old grandson to visit. The first nurse he asked refused, saying it was "against policy" for an underage child to visit patients in ICU. An hour later, he asked a second nurse, who not only granted permission but went to the lobby to fetch the child. The patient died later that night.

"From now on," the chief executive said to all his employees, "I want every one of you to break the rules when necessary to do the 'right' thing for our patients and their families. I trust you to know when to break the rules." He promised to never discipline an employee for using common sense and subsequently created a culture where breaking the rules for the right reasons was cherished.

CHECKLIST FOR A SUCCESSFUL ENGAGEMENT

Healthcare organization leaders may achieve optimal customer service performance without consultants. Some chief executives and department managers can achieve success through setting positive examples and creating the culture in which service excellence thrives. For most organizations, consulting assistance adds value to the pursuit of service excellence. Suggestions for a successful engagement focus on the following.

1. *Instill culture.* Incorporate customer service performance as a permanent aspect of your organization's culture, not a one-time consulting project or passing fad.
2. *Commit.* Be prepared to address problems in facilities, systems, and people. Customer service excellence is not just the organization's culture; it incorporates all aspects of the customer's experience working in concert to achieve optimal service before, during, and after contact with the organization.

3. *Hire wisely.* Use consultants sparingly. Combine consultants' experiences with internal staff's knowledge of customers and processes to develop ideas that will achieve desired customer service results. Select consultants who are able to arrange a visit to a former client who has achieved and sustained optimal customer service performance.

4. *Reward and punish.* Be prepared to reward customer service excellence and punish customer service indifference. Not every employee can be a service star, but those who are truly indifferent or hostile should undergo a change of employment.

5. *Measure results.* Customer service is a dynamic process. Measure ongoing performance so that positive results can be acknowledged and less than optimal results can receive attention for further improvement.

CONCLUSION

Excellent customer service and clinical quality performance are the foundations on which successful healthcare organizations are built. If they are present, excellent financial performance will follow. Leadership is the most important ingredient in achieving excellent customer service. Good leaders who receive quality consulting advice can help an organization achieve its highest customer service performance. When that goal is reached, your organization can then consider how best to market itself, as discussed in the next chapter.

CHAPTER FIFTEEN

Marketing

A N EMINENT MARKETING consultant once told the chief executive of a mediocre healthcare organization, "The worst thing you can do with a poor service is to sell more of it. If you want to make this organization do even more poorly, let's develop a great marketing campaign. If you want to do well in the long run, forget about marketing for now and fix your problems." Although marketing benefits good organizations and those committed to becoming good organizations, it is of limited value to mediocre organizations and may even be harmful.

The marketing process can strengthen the performance of excellent services within a healthcare organization. Properly executed, marketing can boost volume and customer service performance and ultimately lead to improvements in an organization's financial performance.

There are six aspects to marketing a service or organization:

1. Research
2. Objective evaluation
3. Strength building
4. Communication
5. Feedback
6. Refinement

For marketing to be effective, all six components must be present. Some healthcare organization leaders jump straight to communication in their wish to sell a service or an entire organization. Their view of marketing is that it is primarily advertising and promotion. Focusing on communication alone almost inevitably leads to disappointing results.

Emergency Room Backfire: A large urban hospital completed a strategic plan that identified the emergency room service as a weakness, principally because of the outdated facility. The hospital undertook the development of a completely new emergency room, investing $4 million and two years in the project. The new facility expanded the hospital's potential emergency room patient capacity by 50 percent.

Several months before the new facility opened, the hospital, in conjunction with a local advertising agency, planned a comprehensive advertising campaign. Television, radio, and print media ads were developed, highlighting the opening of the state-of-the-art emergency room. The campaign began one month before the ribbon cutting for the new facility. By opening day, it was clear the campaign had worked. Then the hospital became a victim of its advertising success.

During the first month of occupancy of the new facility, patient volume skyrocketed by 30 percent. However, the increase in volume was short-lived. The new emergency room was unprepared for the increased patient traffic. To keep costs down, physician and nurse staffing was kept at the same level as for the old emergency room. Increased volume overwhelmed the staff and average waiting times tripled from one hour to three. Dissatisfaction was rampant. Angry patients told their friends and neighbors to avoid the new emergency room.

During the second month of operation, emergency room patient volume had dropped to 70 percent of the old facility's patient visits. And it stayed there for the next year. The hospital spent the next year fine-tuning staffing and patient flow systems to handle future volume increases. Finally, two years after opening the new emergency room, it gained back the volume it had lost as the result of its premature advertising campaign.

Advertising without the full marketing process behind it can do more harm than good. The objective of this chapter is to identify circumstances where marketing can be strategically beneficial and to evaluate how consultants can compliment internal staff's efforts to market the organization. Consultants are not always necessary to achieve success in marketing—many organizations achieve success by using their internal resources in creative and effective ways.

WHEN A MARKETING CONSULTANT ADDS VALUE

Marketing consultation is a discipline that can help an organization focus its development efforts on matching customer needs with the strengths of the entire organization or a specific service. Marketing consultation brings research prominently to the forefront. Research conducted by marketing consultants can be in the form of focus groups, telephone or written surveys, or personal interviews with customers or potential customers. Research brings objective data to the organization.

Research also brings objectivity to analyzing customer satisfaction data. Consultants can often obtain more critical feedback from customers than organization representatives. Critical feedback is vital to help an organization's leaders understand its true strengths and weaknesses. A hospital's leaders may believe their obstetrics service is a strength because they have fine physicians, excellent nurses, and a brand-new facility. They may be puzzled as to why the number of deliveries is not growing. Marketing consultants may discover that women value flexibility in the birthing experience more than elegance in patient room furnishings. They may discover that the hospital across town has an older facility but offers physicians and nurses with flexible attitudes about the birthing experience. A marketing consultant can objectively assess these types of strengths and weaknesses in an organization and its competitors.

Providing a reality check for strategic direction is another contribution marketing consultants can bring to an organization. A community hospital may make developing its cardiology program a strategic goal. Marketing consultation can provide the organization with an objective, research-based analysis that defines which medical and support services must be improved before cardiology can become a strategic strength. For example, market research may discover that the community views the hospital as caring but old-fashioned. This image must change before cardiology, a high-tech service, can be emphasized.

Potential Fulfilled: A hospital in a large city completed a strategic plan following the hiring of a new chief executive. The strategic plan identified obstetrics as one of the hospital's biggest weaknesses and a potential service for future growth.

Older white residents of European descent had historically populated the hospital's immediate neighborhood. The hospital's clinical services were built around the needs of Medicare patients. However, in the five-year period preceding the strategic plan, the neighborhood had changed dramatically. The elderly residents moved to the suburbs and were replaced by young Hispanic families. Women's health services, primarily obstetrics, were urgently needed, but the hospital had only two obstetricians, neither of whom spoke Spanish. In addition, the obstetrics facilities were outdated and uninviting.

A thorough market research program was undertaken, strengths and weaknesses were identified, and actions implemented to address the weaknesses of the obstetrics department. More modern facilities, Spanish-speaking physicians and nurses, more flexible payment plans, and expanded visiting hours were all determined to be priorities. The hospital worked with its physicians and staff to design a completely new birthing unit to accommodate these priorities. Over a three-year period, the hospital updated facilities and recruited five new obstetricians, three of them fluent in Spanish. One year after the new birthing unit was finished, a comprehensive advertising program was launched, focusing on the physicians. Two years later, the obstetrics business had tripled. In this instance, the hospital, physicians, and the community all benefited from the marketing process.

When the entire marketing process is brought to bear on a strategic initiative, excellent results can follow. Marketing consultants and the framework they bring to an organization can help integrate strategic initiatives with growth and improved financial performance. There are no shortcuts, however. You cannot have a brainstorm, move directly to the advertising stage to promote the new ideas, and expect to succeed. The five steps of research, objective evaluation, strength building, communication, and feedback and refinement must be followed. Of all these steps, communication—in the form of advertising—may be the least important. Having a strong service is the most important. Consultants can be invaluable in helping focus on what is most important first. When consultants can add value to the marketing process, you must define what it is you need to ensure the best consultant is selected.

DEFINING THE ENGAGEMENT SCOPE

A marketing consultation may be narrowly focused on a specific service or broadly focused on the entire organization. Regardless of whether the scope is narrow or broad, defining the consultation scope follows the same pattern. There are five important elements of a marketing consultation:

1. Research
2. SWOT (strength, weakness, opportunity, and threat) analysis
3. Identification of alternative approaches
4. Marketing action plan recommendations
5. Implementation timetable and milestones

The research portion of the scope of services should define the desired research methodologies (for example, focus group, interviews, or telephone sources). It should also define the constituencies to be researched. Typically, it is desirable to research current users of the service or organization, users of competitors' services, potential users, and past users who have migrated to a competitor.

Insights gained during the research phase will be useful in completing the SWOT analysis. Additional insights of the organization's leadership and staff will complement research findings to attain a full appreciation of the strengths and weaknesses of the service or organization.

After completing research and the SWOT analysis, consultants and organization leaders should compile an array of alternate strategies. This is the brainstorming and creative aspect of the marketing consultation process.

After alternatives have been enumerated, consultants and organization leaders should define a marketing action plan. The action plan is a road map of the entire set of actions that should take place to effectively market the service or organization. It should include actions for systems and processes, equipment and facilities, human resources, and communications. Note that the communication action plan plays a supporting role, not the principal role.

The final element of the engagement scope is the implementation schedule and reporting milestones to determine whether or not the marketing action plan is achieving its desired goals.

These five key aspects of the marketing consultation engagement provide the basis for producing a request for proposal (RFP) for consideration by potential marketing consultants. Evaluating the RFP responses is the next step in the consultant selection process.

SELECTING THE BEST MARKETING CONSULTANT

A wide variety of consultants are available for marketing healthcare organizations. Small firms may have several highly experienced principals who use subcontractors for specialty skills such as research and advertising. Medium-size firms offer a full range of marketing services in-house and large marketing and consulting firms often have healthcare marketing divisions. The capabilities of the various alternatives should be sampled when selecting a marketing consultant.

RFPS should be sent to three to five marketing firms. When RFP responses are returned, several important criteria should be used to judge the consultants' capability. First, the firm's knowledge and experience is important. Has the firm performed other marketing consultations for similar organizations that have been successful? Next, the experience of the lead consultant and team of consultants assigned to the engagement is important. The capability of the engagement leader can make the difference between brilliant success and bleak failure.

Research capability is another important criterion. Does the firm have a first class in-house research staff or access to this capability through a subcontractor? Research data will be the foundation of the marketing consultation, so research must be a strength of the firm you are considering.

Methodology used by the firm is another selection criteria. Marketing firms vary widely in their approach to a marketing challenge. You must select a firm whose methodology is compatible with your organization's culture.

Usually the list of final candidates can be narrowed to several good options by applying the above criteria. Reference checks and personal interviews are used to make the final selection. With marketing consultations, as with other kinds of consultations, it is important to check references from client assignments that have had enough time to demonstrate success or failure. Between 6 and 12 months after the marketing action plan is implemented is sufficient time to show a success or failure trend. Also, care should be taken to conduct reference checks on engagements that used the lead consultant who is being proposed for the engagement at your organization.

Finally, personal interviews with the proposed consultation team should be conducted to determine compatibility and chemistry between the parties. After conducting reference checks and personal interviews, the first choice of consultants should be obvious. Once the selection is made, you should conduct final negotiations regarding professional fees and the engagement timetable and prepare a mutually acceptable engagement contract. When the engagement contract is finalized, the focus shifts to preparing for a successful engagement.

PREREQUISITES FOR A SUCCESSFUL CONSULTATION

Marketing is intended to be an organizational commitment, not a short-term fix for an organization's ills. Marketing must be viewed as a process involving research, refining strengths of a service or the entire organization, implementing an action plan, and receiving feedback from customers so that the service or organization can be improved. This level of commitment requires the support of the chief executive if the entire organization is to benefit from marketing or the lead manager if a particular department is to benefit from marketing. Support for the consultation team leader is the first prerequisite for success.

A commitment to conduct research and to pay attention to its findings is the second prerequisite for success. Research findings and the accompanying SWOT analysis indicate what strengths can be promoted and what weaknesses must be fixed. Preparing all of the support systems appropriately prior to marketing is also vital for success. Promoting a program or service ill-prepared for an influx of new customers guarantees disaster.

Marketing should be viewed as a long-term process if it is to be successful. The marketing cycle begins with research and ends with analysis and refinement of results, another form of research. It takes months, sometimes even years, to judge the ultimate success or failure of a particular marketing initiative.

It is important to develop an organizational culture that supports marketing initiatives. It does no good to market a program, such as mammography, if an overworked staff treats every new customer rudely. Unhappy customers will give the program a poor reputation, defeating even the most well-conceived advertising campaign. Marketing may bring new customers, but only the organization's staff and support systems can satisfy and retain these customers.

A successful marketing initiative should have feedback mechanisms to measure results and definitive goals against which to measure progress. Finally, the organization must be prepared to use the feedback it receives to refine the initiative based on actual customer experiences.

PITFALLS TO AVOID DURING A MARKETING CONSULTATION

A pitfall into which many healthcare organizations blunder is marketing an inferior service or program. If volume declines for a clinical service, it is likely that something is wrong with the service. Instead of researching the cause for the decline, some organization leaders believe promoting the service is the solution for the decline. They inevitably fall victim to the rule of marketing that says never sell more of a poor product or service. Fix the problem; then consider marketing.

Along with the tendency to use advertising to fix a declining service, a related tendency is to throw money at problem services. Some chief executives think that if business is slow, full-page ads and television commercials will build it back up. Again, a problem service cannot be fixed by throwing money at it.

Advertising a chief executive's "brainstorm" is not marketing. Marketing, when supported by capable consultants working with a competent leadership team, can achieve great results. Promoting a brainstorm can lead to embarrassment.

> **Fighting Seniors:** A community hospital chief executive was working with a skilled marketing consultant to create a series of new programs for senior citizens. Market research showed that the organization was particularly weak in its services to Medicare patients, so the chief executive was anxious to develop creative programs to serve this population.
>
> The marketing consultant recommended special amenities such as designated parking, assistance with interpreting healthcare bills, transportation, and special scheduling considerations for seniors. During the planning process, the chief executive had a brainstorm, "Why don't we

offer meals to seniors at a 50 percent discount in our cafeteria?" The marketing consultant advised against this. The chief executive didn't listen, however. He was sure his "marketing" brainstorm would be a winner.

When the new senior programs were unveiled, the discounted meals stimulated the most definitive response—unfortunately. Hundreds of seniors descended on the hospital's cafeteria every day. They came in such numbers that employees and physicians could not get service. Seniors fought among themselves for the best tables and elbowed staff members out of the service line. After a few days, the cafeteria was in such pandemonium that the chief executive had to admit defeat and eliminate the discount meal portion of the seniors' amenities. For months afterward, he received angry letters from senior citizens about the elimination of this short-lived benefit. The remainder of the seniors' program never had a chance to succeed.

Chief executives with short attention spans can be another problem. Successful marketing is a long-term organizational commitment. It takes months and sometimes even years to see results of a successful marketing engagement. Short-term fixes simply do not work.

Other healthcare leaders claim to have a "feel" for their customers. They purport to "know their market" and do not wish to have their perceptions contradicted by research. These executives are rarely right about their markets. Whether a consultant or internal resources are used, research is always superior to "feelings."

CHECKLIST FOR A SUCCESSFUL MARKETING EXPERIENCE

Marketing success cannot be achieved by shortcuts and expenditures of insufficient amounts of time and money. Marketing success comes from following these six steps.

1. *Research.* Take the time to do the research. Find out what customers truly think of the organization or service. Find out, too, what non-customers think of competitors' services.
2. *Be objective.* Using research and internal knowledge, complete an objective assessment of strengths and weaknesses. Understand what it will take to enhance strengths and correct problems.

3. *Market only strengths.* Endeavor to market an organization's strengths only. Select a specific program or aspect of the organization that distinguishes itself by its excellence. Never market a poorly performing service.

4. *Adjust and refine.* During and after marketing initiatives, adjust and refine the service based on feedback from customers. Continuously attempt to improve the service.

5. *Measure.* Measure marketing performance based on predetermined goals. If success is not achieved, go back to the research phase to understand why.

6. *Emphasize people.* Marketing success is supported by facilities, technology, and systems, but can only be achieved through people. Superb people can satisfy customers in spite of less-than-optimal facilities and technology. Poorly performing people, or capable people performing with poor attitudes, can never be overcome with good facilities and technology.

MARKETING INITIATIVES WITHOUT CONSULTANTS

Motivated leadership in an organization can succeed with most aspects of marketing without outside consultation. Members of the staff may credibly perform research. Focus groups, customer interviews, and telephone surveys are well within the capability of an organization's leadership. Listening carefully to customers can be accomplished without consultation. Customer hot lines, personal visits to customers by organization leaders, customer surveys, e-mail, and web site access may all be employed without outside assistance. It takes time and commitment, but so does quality marketing consultation.

Communication initiatives may also be implemented without professional assistance. While advertising programs may be best left to professionals, there are many other ways to communicate with potential customers. Physician participation in community events, health fairs and wellness screening programs, and open house events are all excellent vehicles to promote awareness of your services. Interviews and feature stories in local media are also highly effective and cost far less than paid advertising.

Observing best practices in a community and learning from them is another strategy for reducing the need for professional consultation. For example, if a local retailer is well known for extraordinary customer service, a healthcare chief executive could learn from this counterpart in the retail industry. Many excellent marketing initiatives have been duplicated by observant chief executives who transfer a good marketing idea from a non-healthcare setting to his or her healthcare organization.

Some superb healthcare organizations have never needed the services of a marketing consultant. These rare organizations are led by gifted chief executives, physicians, and managers who incorporate marketing into the culture of their organization. For most organizations, however, some professional consultation will enhance marketing success.

CONCLUSION

Marketing must be viewed as a comprehensive process, not a short-term initiative. Marketing success depends on good leadership and on creating excellent programs for customers. It is never just an ad campaign or a quick fix for a poorly functioning service.

Performance of the human resources of an organization, its people, can make or break a marketing program—or an entire organization. Consultation in the human resource arena is the subject of the next chapter.

CHAPTER SIXTEEN

Human Resources

T HE HEALTHCARE BUSINESS is a people business. Hospitals, physician offices, long-term care facilities, clinics, and every other healthcare organization rely on people to render professional services. Technology plays an important supporting role, but people provide the services on which the healthcare industry is based. Human resources are every bit as important as the facilities, high tech equipment, and space-age systems that comprise the healthcare industry.

All healthcare organizations have a human resources function, which encompasses hiring staff, establishing compensation and benefits, creating and administering human resources policies, record keeping, organization development, and overseeing discipline procedures and performance evaluations. Human resources functions are highly regulated and subject to a wide array of local, state, and federal guidelines as well as professional accreditation standards. In organizations like hospitals, major clinics, and long term care facilities, it is common for human resources to be a major department. In smaller organizations like physician offices, human resources functions are usually handled by the office manager.

Healthcare organizations today face extraordinary challenges in the human resources arena. There is an ongoing shortage of qualified professional staff. In some professions, like nursing, the shortage is so acute that an entire new industry—agency staffing—has been created to assist healthcare organizations fill open nursing positions. The extremely high premium charged by these agencies is creating a secondary financial crisis in the hospitals, clinics, and long-term care facilities they service.

The costs of staff recruitment, training, and retention have placed high levels of stress on healthcare organizations, particularly hospitals. In some parts of the country, trained staff must be imported to keep the doors open. In addition, healthcare organizations are operating in an increasingly competitive environment, where the attitude of employees can make the difference between gaining market share or closing the doors forever. All of these factors are leading healthcare organizations to focus more on the human resources function. High-performing healthcare organizations achieve and sustain success partially as a result of recruiting, retaining, and motivating a high-performing staff.

This chapter will help you to:

- identify potential areas of value for human resources consultations;
- encourage thoughtful selection of human resources consultants; and
- articulate alternatives to consultants in several key areas of human resources administration.

WHEN TO RETAIN A HUMAN RESOURCES CONSULTANT

Human resources consultants may be useful to healthcare organizations in three different areas: process, projects, and problem solving. Consultants can help healthcare organizations focus on process improvement, such as hiring, benefit administration, performance evaluation, and policy administration. Consultants may be retained to analyze the strengths and weaknesses of these essential and instrumental processes and to recommend refinements and improvements not evident to internal human resources staff.

Consultants may also be useful with human resource projects that are temporary in nature and usually intended to address a specific human resource challenge. Examples could include compensation strategy, organization development, and cost-reduction initiatives. Consultants may bring valuable insights to these projects, which, when added to the human resources staff's perspectives, may create unique and successful strategies that benefit the organization.

Finally, consultants may be beneficial in addressing human resource problems such as agency staff reliance, union organizing, employee terminations, and legal challenges to disciplinary actions. The list of potential human resources problems is infinite. Although most can be resolved internally, the selective use of experienced consultants can help healthcare organizations save time and money when faced with problems that other organizations have experienced and solved with the help of outside consultants. Knowing when the problem is severe enough to warrant the use of a consultant is a judgment that some organizations are reluctant to make. This reluctance sometimes leads to bigger problems.

Agency Dilemma: A long-term care facility experienced an acute shortage of nursing assistants. During the previous year, resignations and an inability to recruit replacements resulted in a nursing assistant vacancy rate of 50 percent. The director of nursing had no alternative but to begin using agency staff to fill the nursing assistant openings.

Unable to envision a solution to this growing problem, the administrator retained a human resources consultant to review the situation. The consultant comprehensively studied the hiring process, pay and benefits, working conditions, and all aspects of the nursing assistants' role in the facility. The results of the study were enlightening. The consultant found that the principal reason for turnover among nursing assistants was the poor attitude of the nursing staff toward the assistants' work and importance. Nurses were rude and insensitive to the nursing assistants and frequently belittled them in front of residents.

The solution involved attitude adjustment training for the nursing staff. While most nurses responded positively, several resisted changing their negative attitudes. These nurses were subsequently terminated after the organization followed its progressive discipline procedures. After the attitudes of the remaining nursing staff improved, the facility was able to successfully recruit and retain new nursing assistants. Some even came from the ranks of agency nursing assistants. In the final analysis, this human resources challenge was resolved with an adjustment of attitude instead of an adjustment in pay. The consultant played a key role in defining the problem and outlining the solution.

DEFINING THE SCOPE OF THE ENGAGEMENT

As with most consulting assignments, the first and most important step in defining the scope of the engagement is articulating the desired outcome. In the agency dilemma example above, the following issues were defined to determine the scope of the engagement.

1. *Desired outcome.* Eliminate the use of agency nursing assistant staff within 90 days.
2. *Problem:* A 50 percent vacancy rate in nursing assistant positions, forcing the use of agency staff.
3. *Organization resources.* Access to all records, staff interviews, agency staff records, and other documents or records related to the problem.
4. *Accountability.* Consultant to be accountable to director of nursing.
5. *Timeframe.* Consultant study to be completed in 30 days or less.

These five steps helped the director of nurses at the long-term care facility define the scope of the engagement with the human resources consultant. In this instance, the consultant was retained to solve a problem. The same five-step approach should be used if the human resources consultation under consideration is a process improvement challenge or a special project initiative. After defining the scope of the engagement, the selection process for a human resources consultant can begin.

SELECTING THE BEST HUMAN RESOURCE CONSULTANT

A wide variety of excellent human resources consultants are available to healthcare organizations. Several medium-size and large firms exclusively serve healthcare clients in all their consulting needs. Many small and medium-size firms serve healthcare and other service industry human resources clients. In addition, law firms often have expertise available in labor law and other related human resources specialty areas.

Finding excellent human resources consultants is similar to finding other specialty consultants. Some sources for potential consultants include:

- references from professional colleagues who have had good personal experience with the consultant (this is the most valuable referral source);

- human resources professional associations at the state and national levels;
- articles written by consultants in human resources professional journals; and
- professional development conferences with human resources consultants as speakers.

For most healthcare human resources engagements, identifying three to five potential consultants is usually sufficient. Make a pre-qualifying phone call to each firm identified to verify their interest and availability. The pre-qualifying call is also a good source of current contact information for the request for proposal (RFP). After verifying interest, you should prepare a consulting RFP using the general format outlined in the scope of the engagement suggestions discussed above.

When evaluating RFP responses, particular attention should be given to the experience of the proposed consultants to be assigned to the engagement, the firm's ability to meet RFP requirements, and the availability of references with a successful outcome.

Checking references on the best two or three firms based on the RFP responses is the next step in the selection process. The person in the organization who will be responsible for coordinating the engagement should check the consultants' references, preferably by telephone. Achievement of engagement results, quality of the working relationship, and the firm's ability to complete the engagement on time and on budget are the most critical aspects of the reference checks.

Finally, one or two of the best firms should be invited for personal interviews. An interview gives the consultants an opportunity to present their capabilities and their enthusiasm for the engagement. It gives you the opportunity to judge organization compatibility and consulting styles. Following interviews, you should be able to comfortably select the best consultant to meet your organization's needs.

PREREQUISITES FOR A SUCCESSFUL HUMAN RESOURCES CONSULTATION

The first prerequisite for a successful consultation, including a human resources consultation, is the execution of a well-crafted letter of engagement. The letter of engagement for a human resources consultation should follow the general format provided in Appendix G at the end of this book. The letter of engagement sets forth the mutual expectations and goals of the organization and the consultant.

Both the organization and consulting firm must devote the necessary resources to make the engagement a success. For the organization, this means having the time available to work with the consultant. From the consulting firm's perspective, this means having sufficient time to devote to your needs without conflicting time demands from other engagements. If both aspire to the expectations and devote sufficient time and resources, the engagement has a very good chance of succeeding.

During the engagement, both the organization's contact person and the consultant must devote adequate time to communication and updating each other and resolving minor problems that can frequently arise.

At the end of the consultation, the organization's leaders must have the resolve and commitment to follow through on the consultant's recommendations. If the objective of the engagement was well articulated initially and the consultant was selected with appropriate due diligence, it is likely that both the organization and consultant will be satisfied with the engagement outcome. Then it is up to you to implement the consultant's recommendations, which is always the final challenge of any consulting engagement.

> **Hiring Process Overhaul:** A large medical clinic's leaders believed that their hiring process was not performing optimally. The human resources director had strong opinions about the role of her department in the hiring process. Her view of the hiring process was that it was best left to the professionals in her department with minimal input from other departments beyond developing basic job descriptions.
>
> Physicians and managers in the clinic grew uncomfortable with this approach. Some employees were hired who were incompatible with their supervisors. This led to high turnover and dissatisfaction among physicians and managers at the clinic. The clinic administrator and human resources director decided to retain a consultant to give an objective "second opinion" about the centralized hiring process.
>
> After numerous interviews with employees, physicians, and managers, the consultant concluded that the centralized hiring process was functioning very well in identifying qualified candidates for job openings. Where the process seemed to be flawed was that hiring input from the

physician or manager who would be working with the prospective employee was never sought. On a trial basis, human resources began sending two or three qualified candidates for a "final interview" with the physician or manager to solicit their input before a final hiring decision was made. The trial went extremely well, and this new process was adopted as part of the hiring procedure on a permanent basis.

Human resources was pleased because turnover dropped dramatically. Physicians and managers were pleased because they now felt they had a say in the hiring process. And the consultant was pleased because the clinic became an excellent reference for future clients.

Pitfalls to Avoid with a Human Resources Consultant

Human resources consultants can assist healthcare organizations by bringing their objectivity, creativity, and wide-ranging experiences to bear on process improvements, special projects, or problem solving. One thing they cannot and should not be expected to do is solve problems that stem from ineffective or poor management. One common pitfall experienced by organizations is bringing in a human resources consultant to solve a problem that can only be addressed by the organization itself. For example, if the nurse turnover rate in a medical center's intensive care unit is extraordinarily high because the nurse manager is a complete ogre, no amount of consulting creativity will be able to lower the turnover rate unless the nurse manager changes her management style.

Another problem experienced by organizations is accepting a "canned response" from the consultant. Just because something works in Peoria is no guarantee that it will work in Salt Lake City. The consultant should be challenged to deliver recommendations to your unique situation and problems, not simply to dress up approaches that have been tried elsewhere.

A third problem with human resources challenges occurs when an organization fails to recognize situations where consultation may be a positive step. As with other consulting disciplines, organization leaders may not recognize situations in which consultants can add value by solving an intractable problem or helping the organization capitalize on an opportunity for positive change. In rare instances, it takes a figurative slap in the face to wake up an organization's leaders.

Experience

Human resources consultants add value to many challenges faced by healthcare organizations. An extremely wide range of "people" problems and opportunities face healthcare organizations. While no substitute exists for good internal leadership in solving problems or capitalizing on opportunities, the use of consultants can be highly beneficial. Five keys to achieving a successful experience with human resources consultants follow.

1. *Define.* Define the problem to be solved or the opportunity to improve clearly. Articulate the desired outcome from the consultation.
2. *Resources.* Line up the necessary internal resources to support the consultation. Be sure the right people are available to assist the consultants.
3. *Select.* Select the best human resources consultant available. Look for experience and the ability to help the organization make and sustain changes.
4. *Unique solution.* Make the solution or strategy unique to the organization. Never settle for a "cookie cutter" response or program.
5. *Implement.* Implement the consultant's recommendations and then follow through to be sure the solution achieved the intended outcome.

Alternatives to Consultants

While the use of human resources consultants can be very positive, some human resources challenges can be well handled by the use of internal resources. One typical assignment for human resources consultations is to perform an employee attitude survey. These surveys can be invaluable for identifying problems with management or organization culture. Human resources consultants can bring expertise and objectivity to these surveys. On the other hand, human resources departments are in an excellent position to work with senior management to perform these kinds of surveys internally. Human resources professionals can construct the survey questions and senior management can encourage employees to participate in the anonymous survey by promising to accurately and objectively present the results to the staff after the surveys have been completed and then acting on the results. Human resources professionals can summarize survey results and highlight issues for further consideration by senior management.

Performing compensation surveys is another function for which human resources consultants are often called on to assist healthcare organizations. As an alternative, the human resources staff can formulate survey questions and personally telephone their counterparts in comparative organizations. Promising to share the survey results usually encourages enough participation to make the survey results valuable. The availability of compensation data on-line also makes it reasonable for many of these surveys to be conducted without extensive consulting help.

The application of common sense and high leadership standards to human resources problems is another area where healthcare organizations can potentially forego human resources consultations. When a problem occurs, even a big one, the organization's leaders should first consider their own response before quickly retaining a consultant. Leaders should try to understand the origin of the problem without becoming defensive or prematurely making a judgment. Often, human resources problems are symptomatic of larger organization culture problems that require thoughtful solutions instead of quick fixes.

Brawl in the Records Room: A prominent internal medicine specialist investigated loud noises coming from the medical records room of his office and discovered two of his office staff engaged in a fistfight. While breaking up the fight, he received a punch in the nose.

The physician had sold his medical practice to the local hospital he and his father had practiced in for 50 years. After the sale, his staff no longer reported to or was accountable to him. Instead, they reported to the "corporate practice manager" located in an office building 10 miles away. After stopping his nose bleed, the physician called the corporate office for help. He got voice mail, instructing him to leave a message.

The physician returned to the medical records room and promptly fired the two employees who had been fighting. Hours later, when the corporate practice manager returned the physician's call, the firing was overturned, and employees were reinstated after a one-day suspension. The physician protested but was told that the program of progressive discipline followed by the practice management policies required suspension before firing, no matter how bad the offense. The physician again protested and was told that if he did not like the human resources policy, he could seek employment elsewhere. Because of this and other frustrations, he subsequently did just that. He moved his practice to a new location and started over again. He made sure that he retained hiring and firing power in his new office.

Could a consultant have helped this situation? Probably not. What could have helped were a dose of common sense and a higher level of standards from the practice management corporation. When employees get into fistfights, they should be discharged, period. Following a well-intended progressive discipline policy is no excuse for retaining employees who should be terminated.

CONCLUSION

Healthcare organizations large and small can benefit from the thoughtful use of human resources consultants. As with any other consultation, you must articulate the problem and desired outcome before retaining the consultants. Human resources consultants cannot be expected to substitute for common sense and high standards of management performance.

No less demanding than human resources challenges are those of designing and building the optimal physical facilities for healthcare operations. Selecting the best architect is the subject of the next chapter.

CHAPTER SEVENTEEN

Architects

O NE OF THE most exciting opportunities for any healthcare organization chief executive officer and senior management team is planning a new facility or extensive renovation of an existing facility. Creating new "bricks and mortar" has an allure that many leadership teams have not had the opportunity to experience. However, hospital and healthcare facilities built in the 1950s and 1960s with government funding programs such as the Hill-Burton Act will soon need complete updating or replacement. More healthcare organization leaders will experience the exhilaration and the exasperation of creating new facilities. They will share these experiences with their consultants: architects.

The challenge of creating a new facility or renovating an existing one is composed of several related goals. Creating the absolute best facility for the community and customer is one goal. Creating a facility that is functional for its users is also highly desirable, as is creating a facility that is beautiful. Creating a facility that is efficient for the staff who work within its walls is another goal. Creating a facility that fits within the organization's budget is a necessity.

An architect is the principal consultant for creating new or renovated healthcare facilities. Engineers, facility planners, interior design specialists, and a host of other experts also contribute, but the architect is the central leader of the consulting team. The selection of and working relationship with the architect determines whether a facility meets and possibly even exceeds its expectations. The selection of the right architect can assist the healthcare organization in creating a functional, beautiful, and

efficient facility. The selection of the wrong architect can lead to an un-
appealing, inefficient, and costly mistake. Unfortunately, these mistakes
are not easily undone once bricks and mortar have been set in place.

This chapter is devoted to explaining the issues surrounding selecting and working with architects when a new facility is being planned, or
a major ($2 million plus) renovation on an existing facility is being con-
templated. Smaller projects may not need an architect. For healthcare
chief executives, selecting an architect may be a once-in-a-professional-
lifetime opportunity. The thrill of leading the development of a new facility is incomparable, a lasting tribute to a successful leadership tenure.
Care must be taken, however, that it is not a career-ending project.

ARCHITECTS AND THE FACILITIES PLANNING TEAM

All facility replacement or renovation decisions should be preceded by a
sound strategic plan. When a new, renovated, or extensively remodeled
facility is necessary to achieve a strategic goal, it is essential to engage an
architect.

The first step in the selection process is to understand the role of the
architect. Architects are responsible for the overall design, exterior and
interior, of the facility. But their work involves much more. Engineering,
selection of construction materials and methodologies, site planning,
building systems, and design of interior spaces are all part of the architect's purview. Often, architects also are involved in the equipment selection and interior design.

On some healthcare organization facilities projects, facilities planning
consultants are also an integral part of the consulting team. These facilities planners are healthcare experts who are experienced in assisting
architectural firms and healthcare organizations design optimal facility
layouts to best meet their needs. For example, facilities planners with
healthcare expertise can help create efficient, functional layouts and
workspaces. Their in-depth knowledge of how healthcare organizations
work can help architects plan more effectively for the interrelationships
within facilities. Facilities planners bring a practical planning perspective to the facilities project, complementing the architect's overall design
expertise. Sometimes facilities planning consultants work directly for the
architectural firm; if not, they are also available from consulting firms
that specialize in facilities planning.

There are other important consultants who are part of any facility development project. Financial planners play a role in lining up financial resources to pay for the project. Construction experts are called upon to provide advice on building the project. A range of engineering and other specialties is also available as necessary.

When a facility project is contemplated, the process begins with selecting an architect. Other consultants may be retained, depending on the size of the project and the capabilities of the architect selected, but the architect is the overall consultant who guides the process.

DEFINING THE ENGAGEMENT SCOPE

Hiring an architect is like selecting an internal medicine physician as your primary care doctor. You choose a superb doctor, but you recognize that it may be necessary for specialists to be brought in when their expertise is required. Your internist may ask you to see a cardiologist, an exercise physiologist, or a nutritionist if he is concerned about certain risk factors. No matter what specialists may be appropriate from time to time, you still view the internist as your primary physician. You trust that he or she will get special expertise when needed, but you give the internist responsibility for your overall care.

When defining the scope of the architect's engagement, it is the organization leaders' job to define what is needed. The architect's job is to assemble the appropriate team of experts to meet those needs. For developing a new facility or making major renovations to an existing facility, the following general scope of the engagement is pertinent to healthcare architect selection.

1. *Research.* The architect should review the strategic reasons for developing the new or renovated facility to determine if there are any unanswered questions concerning the basic needs analysis. In addition, the architect should thoroughly research the regulatory environment to determine if there are circumstances that could preclude moving ahead with the facilities project.
2. *Program.* The architect should thoroughly research all of the needed functions of the planned facility to determine the overall size and configuration of the project. Creating a design program— a schematic drawing showing the relative locations of key

services—should entail extensive interviews with facility users to assemble a preliminary layout plan for the facility.

3. *Design.* The architect should be assigned overall responsibility for the facility design, which includes a site plan, exterior building design, interior layouts, and systems design. The design phase follows the program phase and includes the detailed design of the facility and all related systems.

4. *Design tests.* Following the design phase, the architect should "test" key aspects of the design. For example, if a new inpatient wing is being designed, a mock-up of a patient room should be built for detailed examination by the staff who will be working in the room. Although testing the design with mock-ups is rarely done, it is a very desirable step to refine the design and eliminate potential problems with the design or related equipment.

5. *Document preparation.* The architect should prepare detailed construction documents, blueprints, and specifications following the completion of the design and design test phases. These should also include documents to solicit construction bids from contractors.

6. *Bid phase.* The architect should assist organization leaders with soliciting construction bids, analyzing bid responses, and selecting the construction firm and related factors. This should also include preparing a list of construction companies qualified to bid on the project.

7. *Construction oversight.* The architect should assist organization leaders with overseeing construction or renovation of the facility and verify that all construction is consistent with design specifications.

8. *Post-construction test.* The architect should assist organization leaders with testing all facilities and systems following construction to verify that construction and all systems perform according to the design specifications.

9. *Functional review.* Six to twelve months after the new facility becomes operational, the architect should conduct a functional review of how the facility performs against its design goals. This functional review can be very useful as a learning experience for the architect and may result in some modifications to the facility to ensure design goals are met.

This nine-step scope can be inserted into the general request for proposal (RFP) format presented in Appendix H at the end of this book to form the basis of an RFP for architects. While the need for all nine steps may not seem obvious, all of the steps contribute to selecting and working effectively with the best architect and avoiding costly mistakes.

> **Doorway Disaster:** A university hospital undertook a major facility project to replace a two-story inpatient wing. The wing, over 40 years old, was very inefficient for the nursing staff, and the patient rooms were too small to accommodate modern equipment.
>
> The university retained a well-known architectural firm to design the new wing. Although the firm did not have healthcare experience, it was renowned for its design of university facilities. The architects designed the new wing with extensive input from physicians, nurses, and other staff members. Even patients were consulted about the layout of the new rooms. The design was finalized and construction began soon thereafter. Although 100 new patient rooms were to be built, no mock-ups were made to test their layout and efficiency. As construction proceeded, the purchasing department ordered patient beds and other furniture and equipment to be used in the new patient wing.
>
> Several weeks prior to occupying the new building, it was decided to set up a new patient room so the staff could see the layout, furniture, and equipment. It was then that embarrassed project leaders discovered that the new patient beds would not fit through the doorways of the patient rooms. The beds were two inches too wide, or the doorways were two inches too narrow, depending on who was speaking. A finger-pointing session of epic proportions ensued. Ordering narrower beds or widening and replacing the doorframes was going to be very expensive.
>
> After consideration of the options, it was decided to widen the doors of all 100 patient rooms. Opening of the new wing was delayed for months and hundreds of thousands of dollars were spent fixing the problem.
>
> If a mock patient room had been built for a few thousand dollars, this huge mistake could have been avoided. So could the lawsuits that followed this architectural disaster.

SELECTING THE BEST ARCHITECT

Healthcare organizations can choose from many superb architects. The challenge is to narrow the options to a manageable number of choices.

The obvious starting point is architects who have done excellent work for other healthcare facilities in the area. Even in a small community with few healthcare facilities, there may be local architects who could work with healthcare facilities planners to form an outstanding design team. Regional and national healthcare architectural associations can make references. Large healthcare consulting firms also are an excellent source of architect referrals. Healthcare professional journals often feature design reviews and articles written by architects. Finally, architects are often featured speakers at professional development education seminars.

Creating a list of five to ten qualified architects is the starting point for a thorough selection process. Preliminary calls should be made to these firms to determine their initial interest in being considered and their expertise related to the upcoming facility project. Try to narrow the list to about five qualified and interested architects for the RFP phase. Have a mix of different sized architectural firms on the RFP list, ranging from a highly regarded small firm, to several medium-sized firms, to perhaps one or two large firms.

The RFP for architects should be developed using the scope of the engagement section previously discussed integrated with the general RFP format presented in Appendix H at the end of this book. The background section of the RFP should be enhanced with discussion of the strategic reasons for the facility project and details of the current facility such as age, design factors, and reasons for replacement or renovation. In addition, the RFP for architects should require that all prospective firms make a site visit to the facility before submitting the RFP. Site visits should give the architect a better understanding of the facility challenges to be addressed.

Once the RFPs have been released and returned, you are faced with selecting the best architect to meet your organization's needs. There is no substitute for a combination of thorough reference checks and site visits to help make this important decision.

REFERENCE CHECKS AND PERSONAL SITE VISITS

If you were to commission a portrait of your children, the deciding factor in your selection of the artist would be the one whose work you admire most. Of course, price, time to complete, and medium are also important.

But if it is a work of art you want, you will pick an artist whose work you admire. The same is true for an architect.

In reviewing the RFP responses from architects, pay particular attention to the designation of the lead architect, staff to be assigned to your project, past experience with similar facilities, and, of course, references. Personal telephone references are essential and should give you a good perspective on the architect's track record. The absence of excellent client references is a disqualifying factor. RFP reviews and reference checks should allow you to select two or three top choices. Then, ask each prospective architect for facility projects that best represent his or her capability to complete your organization's project. In other words, ask the prospective architect the names of the projects of which he or she is most proud. When one or two projects are identified, a team from the healthcare organization should go to those facilities and spend time personally talking to the leaders who worked with the architect.

These site visits are absolutely invaluable and essential to making an informed choice of architect. They are worth the time, effort, and trip to gain firsthand insights into the capabilities of the architects under consideration. Ask these former clients if they are completely satisfied. Ask what they would do differently with all the benefits of hindsight. Ask if they would hire the same architect again. Asking good questions and making personal observations should give you the knowledge to choose the architect who can best meet your organization's needs. If an architect cannot direct you to a past project he or she is proud of and the client was pleased with, keep looking. On the other hand, if you are thrilled to see the past work of an architect under consideration and visiting with that organization's leaders convinces you that their architect is the best, you know you have found your architect.

PITFALLS TO AVOID WITH ARCHITECTS

Numerous pitfalls exist that should be carefully avoided in selecting and working with architects. You should be especially careful to select an architect who will be a good listener. Ideally, a facility design should be the result of the synergy between a talented and creative architect and input and ideas from a well-informed and articulate client. The architect cannot do his or her best work without input. Unfortunately, some architects are better listeners than others. The reference checking process and site visits should enable you to tell the difference.

Architect arrogance is another danger. Some architects put aesthetic considerations above all else, including functionality and cost. It is highly desirable to have a beautiful facility, but it is even better to have a facility that is both beautiful and functional. Not all architects are equally adept at creating this synergistic combination.

Another pitfall to avoid with architects and facility projects in general is absolute trust in paper plans. Few healthcare professionals are skilled at reading blueprints and visualizing how the design will work. The newest computer design processes enable architects to create three-dimensional, virtual reality presentations that can be very useful. In addition, mock-ups are very useful in testing the functionality of a design before it is actually constructed.

Organization leaders should also insist on original work when they retain architects. Recycling past designs is sometimes a failing of architects. Each facility and its challenges are unique and should warrant a unique architectural design. Nor should you insist on re-creating a design that has proven acceptable in the past. Both parties should begin a facility design project with a fresh perspective.

Organization leaders should also be careful to avoid trying to do the architect's job. Some clients are so aggressively opinionated that even the best architect cannot get a creative thought in edgewise. Clients should never try to displace the architect's contributions with their own opinions, no matter how strongly held. To paraphrase the legal profession, the person who acts as his own architect has a fool for a client.

Finally, both you and your architect should be careful not to use the newest technology or the latest design fad merely to be able to boast that the facility is "state of the art." Such thinking can lead to costly mistakes and disappointments.

Gimmicks and Gizmos: A community hospital opened its doors touting itself as "state of the art." One of the most anticipated technological improvements was a completely automated tray delivery system for all patient meals. Since cold meals are a well-known hospital problem, architects, facilities planners, and food service engineers were determined to solve the problem with the latest technology.

The system they designed was a conceptual marvel. After meal trays were assembled in a centralized kitchen, they were loaded in a robot delivery cart that traversed the hospital via special elevators and hallway monorails. The concept was to speed meals to nursing units where waiting staff would deliver them hot and fresh to patients. Soon after opening, however, the number of complaints about cold food was higher than in the old hospital.

After investigation, it was discovered that the robot food carts frequently got lost and went to the wrong nursing units. Also, they traveled very slowly on the hallway monorails, much slower than a "human-powered" cart. The system was so subject to breakdowns that new employees had to be hired to follow the robot carts to be sure they reached their destinations. Nearly every patient was getting cold meals as a result of these problems.

Finally, the food service manager turned off the robot system and started delivering meal trays using food service personnel. Immediately, complaints about cold food ceased. The hospital discovered in the process that going back to the "old-fashioned" delivery system of walking the tray carts to the nursing units took less than half the time the robot carts did, even when the robots managed to go to the right delivery location. The state-of-the-art food delivery system is gathering dust, but the patients are finally getting hot meals. Bright idea, dim result.

CHECKLIST FOR A SUCCESSFUL ARCHITECTURAL EXPERIENCE

The design and creation of a new facility or an extensively renovated older facility can be a crowning career achievement. The selection of the best architect is a decisive factor in how positive this experience will be. A successful experience is based on the following steps.

1. *Identify the need.* Contemplate a new or renovated facility only based on a strategic need, preferably identified as part of a thoughtful strategic plan.
2. *Define the scope.* Clearly define the scope and expectations of what is desired from the architect. Preliminary research is essential.
3. *Hire the best.* Retain the best architect possible for your project. Find out who is the best by selecting the architect from a qualified group of candidates using a well-written RFP, checking references

carefully, and making site visits to observe the prospective architect's work firsthand.

4. *Test, test, test.* Work with your architect to constantly test assumptions and designs throughout the process. Never rely solely on blueprints. Build mock-ups, try out sample equipment, and frequently ask the opinion of customers and users.

5. *Test again.* After the facility is completed, be sure you and your architect conduct post-construction interviews and further tests to determine if the design is working properly. Make changes and refinements as necessary. Designs are rarely perfect; so do not be afraid to fine-tune them when the facility is open for business.

CONCLUSION

The architect is one of the most important consultants a chief executive will ever engage. It is extraordinarily important to select wisely—the right choice can help achieve the organization's strategic goals. The creation of a new facility or complete renovation of an older facility leaves a lasting legacy that can benefit the organization for decades into the future.

Facilities alone do not make a healthcare organization function as desired. The appropriate selection and deployment of technology is another key factor. The challenges of technology are discussed in the next chapter.

CHAPTER EIGHTEEN

Technology

TECHNOLOGY IS AN impossible subject to write about. Before the ink is dry, the words have become obsolete. Using consultants to help your healthcare organization with its complex and comprehensive technological needs is no less subject to these laws of obsolescence. Unlike turnarounds, financial audits, and strategic planning, technology consulting by its very nature is so fast-changing that no written advice is likely to do the subject justice. So rapid is the pace of technological change that even on-line or real-time consultation available through cyberspace sources is unlikely to keep up.

The objective of this chapter is to briefly explore technology consultation options and their compelling strengths and limitations. Even more important is considering when to pursue technological advancements. No journal article, chapter, or book can hope to assist a healthcare organization leader make a complex technological decision. This chapter is intended, therefore, to help healthcare leaders ask themselves the right questions to find the right solution to fit their technology needs.

TECHNOLOGY CONSULTING OPTIONS

Healthcare organizations use a wide range of technology from communications to medical equipment to information systems to facilities support. Technology used to diagnose and treat illnesses and run the complex enterprises that support these efforts is literally endless. So how do healthcare organizations keep up? To whom do you turn for advice in selecting the appropriate technology for your mission? Several sound options are unlikely to disappear any time soon; technology specialists, major consulting firms, the "big five" accounting firms, and technology companies themselves all offer consultation services to healthcare organizations. Organization leaders conducting their own research can be a viable alternative to technology consultants.

Technology Specialists

In all areas of technology, specialty consulting firms exist that can assist healthcare organization leaders in making decisions. These firms are usually small and highly focused on one particular kind of technological expertise. They can be an excellent option for healthcare organization leaders who desire to upgrade an existing technology where the choice of manufacturers is extensive.

Reviewing technology journal articles, web sites, and advertisements can identify specialty technology firms. Another excellent source is visiting major technology trade shows. Finally, the technology manufacturers themselves may be able to recommend consultants, although their objectivity may be questionable. The great strength of technology specialists is their current and focused knowledge base. These firms usually have available the very best experts in their respective technology fields. On the other hand, turnover of such experts can be extraordinarily high. The challenge faced by healthcare organizations is finding the best consultant in the best specialty firm.

Consulting Giants

All of the major management consulting firms have technology divisions or subsidiary firms with a wide array of technology experience. It is sometimes a challenge to find both technology expertise and healthcare expertise, but major firms have such extensive technological depth that it is reasonable to expect that they can offer up-to-date counsel to healthcare organizations in most areas of technology.

Locating the major firms is not a challenge. They have offices in most metropolitan areas throughout the country. Many of these firms provide "turnkey" consulting services in technology, in which they take the client through all stages, from design through completion, of a project. For example, they may offer system design, hardware selection, and installation startup. Their strongest area of capability often is in the information technology area. Consulting giants often have close ties to technology companies and a wide variety of clients with technology experience. The extensive knowledge base of these large firms enables them to provide excellent technology consultation to healthcare organizations.

"Big Five" Firms

All of the "big five" accounting firms have strong technology capabilities, especially information technology. Information technology consulting has become so big in terms of consulting revenue that several firms have spun off their technology consulting into separate companies. Healthcare organizations in need of information technology consultation often turn to one of the "big five" firms.

These firms also provide a range of technology service from consulting to system design to implementation. In the information technology area, they too offer turnkey services from design through implementation.

Technology Manufacturers

Most manufacturers of technological equipment for the healthcare industry have consulting capability to assist current and prospective customers successfully employ their products. On the one hand, this option offers a very high level of expertise for a specific product. On the other hand, objectivity and consideration of other products may be limited.

This option is an excellent choice if a particular technology has already been selected and there is a leading or dominant manufacturer. The technological expertise available to assist the healthcare organization may be far superior to that of a consulting firm.

Internal Research

For healthcare organization leaders contemplating technology changes, there is no substitute for knowledgeable internal staff researching the available options. If a medical technology is to be updated, for example, the physicians and management leaders responsible for the upgrade should become technology "experts" before making final decisions. Today, much information is available on-line and by contacting existing users of the technology under consideration.

Sometimes it is better to spend the time and energy on site visits to organizations that already use the technology being contemplated than to engage consultants in this fast-changing field. Learning from the positive and negative experiences of other organizations can help you make an important technology decision. Manufacturers are the best sources of such users. They are likely to be very interested in providing locations where their recent technology is being successfully used. If they cannot provide such references, perhaps it is because there are not any successful users yet.

PEOPLE FACTOR

Regardless of the sophistication of the technology under consideration, at some point the effect on the users, that is, the people factor, should be contemplated. In their rush to employ the latest technology, some healthcare organizations do not give nearly enough consideration to this practical subject.

Several considerations are relevant for most healthcare technologies.

1. *Operation.* Who will operate the equipment? Do we have the physicians, staff, and technicians who know how or can be trained to run the equipment?
2. *Repairs.* Who will fix the equipment? When breakdowns inevitably occur, how will we get the equipment repaired? How long will repairs take? What will we do in the interim?
3. *Compatibility.* Will the new technology interface with existing equipment? If not, what ripple effect changes will be necessary to make the new technology function to its full capacity?

More than one new piece of healthcare technology is sitting idle at this moment because no one is around to run it, fix it, or interface it with existing technology. These are the kinds of practical issues that can be best explored by making site visits to organizations that already use the technology. Learn from other people's experiences.

SUCCESSFUL TECHNOLOGY EXPERIENCE

Healthcare organizations are constantly challenged to have the latest and most modern technology in all aspects of their operation. Ultimately, the application of technology becomes as much a philosophical decision as a technology decision.

Unless your organization is a leading-edge research facility, the need to have the absolute latest of every conceivable technology is highly questionable. In general, it is not necessarily a positive experience to be the first with a new technology, the first customer for a new product, or the first client of a technology company.

Healthcare organizations should employ technology to meet strategic objectives. They should not seek to be first with all new technological breakthroughs. That should be left to the research institutions.

CHECKLIST FOR A SUCCESSFUL TECHNOLOGY CONSULTATION

Technology decisions are among the most challenging faced by healthcare organization leaders. Making a decision to upgrade an existing technology or introduce a new technology can be enormously expensive and have far-reaching implications. There is no easy path for technology decisions. Suggestions for making sound decisions include the following:

1. *Define the objective:* Careful consideration of the desired objective for any technology decision should be undertaken. The objective should be consistent with overall organization objectives and be measurable.
2. *Evaluate options:* Before making any technology decision, a full range of options should be considered. Maintaining existing

technology, especially if it is serving the organization well, should always be an option.

3. *Confirm integration:* Verify that the technology under consideration can be successfully integrated into other existing systems in the organization.

4. *Verify:* Verify that the technology under consideration is actually working in similar operations. Do not rely on manufacturer's claims. Go see the technology in action. Talk to users, customers, and support personnel.

5. *Accept second place:* Let other organizations be first with new technology. In technology, being second almost always means the technology works better.

CONCLUSION

Most healthcare organizations should seek to use technology that has already proven itself. Selecting such technologies can be accomplished with good internal research and does not necessarily require heavy expenditures of consulting dollars. If consultation becomes necessary, select the best consultant available with the most current technology expertise.

No matter how good the medical technology, physicians lead the teams using technology for the benefit of healthcare organizations and their patients. Medical staff consultation is the subject of the next chapter.

CHAPTER NINETEEN

Medical Staff Consultants

A HEALTHCARE ORGANIZATION is tied inexorably to its physicians and medical or professional staffs. Consultants may be necessary from time to time, but it has been my experience that medical staffs in general and physicians individually are rarely enthusiastic about the subject of retaining consultants. Perhaps it is the nature of individual physicians to resist the concept of second opinions and the nature of medical staff organizations to guard their independence from uninvited interference.

Nevertheless, medical staff consultants can be extremely useful to healthcare organizations with advice to medical staffs, individual physicians, and management. First, consultants may be useful in advising medical staffs in the areas of quality, utilization, and regulatory compliance. Consultants can also be useful in helping individual physicians with quality, utilization, and behavior problems. Lastly, consultants can be useful in advising healthcare organization leaders on strategic physician matters such as hospital and physician practices, managed care strategies, and developing hospital and physician joint ventures.

Most often medical staff consultants working with healthcare organizations in these three areas are physicians themselves. To be effective in working with medical staffs and physicians, it is beneficial to be a physician. However, a physician's credentials are not enough to be effective. These consultants must have all of the other consulting skills that have been discussed in previous chapters as well. Unfortunately, there is not an abundance of excellent consultants to meet the needs of medical staffs, physicians, and their organization leaders.

The objective of this chapter is to explore the need for consultants in the medical staff and individual physician area, including clarifying needs, defining the consultation scope, and selecting the best consultant. Finally, this chapter will explore the prerequisites that must be present for a successful consultation to take place and a successful outcome to follow.

IDENTIFYING THE NEED FOR MEDICAL CONSULTATION

Medical staff consultants can influence a healthcare organization's quality, behavior, and financial performance. In the area of quality, consultation is most useful when rendered to the entire medical staff organization. For example, the following areas of responsibility apply to medical staffs of hospitals, clinics, and long-term care facilities:

- Credentialing and privileging
- Reappointment
- Performance improvement
- Utilization management

These responsibilities, among others, are usually prescribed by the medical staff's bylaws. Medical staffs are legally accountable to their organization's governing board. Doing an excellent job in these four areas can be problematic for medical staffs. Credentialing new members of the medical staff or granting privileges is sometimes done in a superficial manner, allowing less than stellar physicians to be appointed. Reappointment can be even more problematic and is often a matter of a few perfunctory requirements. Quality assurance, while arguably one of the most important functions of any medical staff, is also arguably one of the most neglected. Utilization management, a blend of quality and economics, is an unusually sensitive area for medical staffs. Less than optimal performance in any one of these four important areas is a motivating factor for a healthcare organization to consider retaining a medical staff consultant.

In the behavior area, consultants can help address individual physician problems. A physician who cuts corners in patient care or has utilization patterns far outside recognized norms could benefit from focused consultation. Some physicians are also known to be substance abusers or have other psychological problems, and counseling by an objective outside consultant may be highly effective. Physicians sometimes have problems controlling their tempers, which can affect the staff and patients in a negative manner. If destructive or inappropriate behavior or poor clinical practice patterns are permitted, the overall organization will eventually suffer.

Finally, medical staff consultants may be useful in areas concerning finances. It is common for hospitals to acquire physician practices or recruit employed physicians. Unfortunately, many of these owned practices have proven to be financial disasters for the hospitals. Consultants may be successful in working with physicians and hospitals to minimize or eliminate the losses. Formulating an effective managed care strategy is very important to both clinics and hospitals. Some consultants are experts in this area. Additionally, it has become common for healthcare organizations and physicians to form joint ventures. Again, consultants may be useful in establishing successful partnerships. It is worthwhile to note that not all of the medical staff consultants who specialize in financial matters are physicians.

Healthcare organization leaders need only to ask themselves three basic questions to determine whether or not medical staff consultants could be useful:

1. *Quality.* Am I completely confident that every member of my medical staff was appointed, credentialed and privileged appropriately, and continues to be competent in every area where he or she has privileges?
2. *Behavior.* Are there any members of my medical staff whose behavior is hurting the quality of care for my patients or the quality of the work environment for my staff?
3. *Finances.* Am I completely satisfied that my staff and I have all the answers when it comes to making our owned physician practices financially viable?

Most healthcare leaders would have to answer one or more of these questions in the negative. The irony is that these medical staff areas have a need for consultation but rarely receive the attention they deserve.

Terminal Denial: The length of stay for Medicare patients at a struggling inner-city hospital was among the highest in the region. Administrators had on many occasions pointed this out to physician leaders of the medical staff and had received what they considered to be superficial responses. The medical staff leadership felt that administration was picking on them and that length of stay was not as bad as administration thought. "We're doing the best we can" was their typical response.

After several years of finger pointing, both the administrator and the medical staff were in for a very rude awakening. The largest HMO serving Medicare patients conducted a study of length of stay patterns for Medicare patients and decided that neither the hospital nor its medical staff was capable of making constructive changes. It effectively fired the hospital and the medical staff by eliminating them as providers for the HMO.

The result was devastating. The hospital lost one-third of its Medicare patients overnight. About one-quarter of the physicians at the hospital lost their largely HMO Medicare practices. After years of denying they had a problem, the medical staff and hospital suffered greatly. If they had worked together before the momentous HMO decision, perhaps they could have reduced the Medicare patient length of stay and avoided the sanction. An objective outside medical staff consultant could have helped both parties.

DEFINING THE SCOPE OF THE ENGAGEMENT

Articulating the desired outcome is the first step in defining the scope of a medical staff consultation. Each of the three kinds of medical staff consultations (quality, behavior, and finances) has some unique characteristics. An example scope of engagement for each type of consultation is shown below.

Quality—Evaluate the physician reappointment process and improve performance.
- *Current system.* Thoroughly understand the current physician reappointment process, including identifying key strengths and weaknesses.

- *Current physicians.* Evaluate the credentials of current physicians and all privileges assigned to them for appropriateness based on quality standards.
- *Options.* Develop comprehensive options to improve the reappointment process.
- *Recommendations.* Develop recommendations to achieve the goal of improving the reappointment process.
- *Action plan.* Prepare an action plan with specific steps, timetable, and accountability to implement recommended improvements.

Behavior—Evaluate claims that Dr. John Smith is verbally abusive to the nursing staff.
- *Background review.* Review all documentation of the alleged behavior problem. Interview Dr. Smith, nursing staff he works with, and administrative and medical staff leaders to whom Dr. Smith is accountable.
- *Findings.* Review findings of records review and interviews with Dr. Smith and administrative, nursing, and medical staff leaders. Invite comments and input on findings.
- *Action plan.* Prepare an action plan to modify abusive behavior and include counseling and periodic follow-up reports to administration and medical staff leaders.
- *Follow-up.* Conduct follow-up records review and interviews three to six months after the consultation.

Finances—Review physician compensation program for employed physician practices and develop strategy to eliminate financial losses.
- *Current agreements.* Review compensation agreements or contracts to become familiar with current practices.
- *Regional norms.* Conduct surveys to determine regional norms and ranges for employed physician practices. Determine variances, if any, between current practice and regional norms.
- *Brainstorming.* Engage employed physicians in brainstorming sessions to gain their input and ideas on potential changes in compensation practices that may successfully return the practices to profitability.

- *Legal review.* Conduct legal review of compensation options developed in brainstorming sessions and identify any legal or regulatory compliance issues.
- *Options.* Develop a range of options that could potentially improve compensation programs and contribute to achieving the goal of returning practices to financial profitability.
- *Consensus.* Achieve consensus buy-in among physicians about which strategies will be most palatable while achieving the objectives.
- *Implementation and communication.* Prepare implementation action plan, timetable, and communication plan to ensure that all parties understand the compensation plan changes and are committed to its successful implementation.

Regardless of whether the medical staff consultation is in the area of quality, behavior, or finance, articulating the scope of the engagement is an excellent first step in achieving a successful result. Failure to think through each of the necessary steps in the scope of the engagement could compromise the end result of the consultation.

Revolt in the Ranks: A large medical practice was losing money and recognized the need for making a change in the way it compensated physicians. Some junior physicians worked extraordinarily hard for what they perceived as low salaries, while other, more senior physicians worked fewer hours for comparatively high salaries. Changes were needed. The clinic's president retained a well-known physician compensation consultant to help craft a new system of compensation.

The consultant researched current agreements and regional norms, brainstormed potential changes, and, after a legal review, developed new compensation options. That was where the consultation stopped. The consultant and clinic president selected a strategy that they favored and announced the changes would be made in thirty days. They failed to build consensus among physicians, and they failed to create a communication plan to effect the proposed changes. Instead, they simply announced the new system.

The results of leaving out these two crucial steps were very detrimental. One-quarter of the clinic physicians quit and took their practices elsewhere. The clinic president was voted out of office, and a new compensation consultant was retained to start the process all over again.

SELECTING THE BEST MEDICAL STAFF CONSULTANT

Medical staff consultants are not nearly as available to healthcare organizations as financial consultants, management consultants, or architects. One option is large consulting and financial services firms with medical staff consultants on staff. Additional options are practicing physicians with part-time consulting practices and small consulting firms that specialize in medical staff matters.

To find consultant alternatives, start with area medical schools or university hospitals. The chancellor's office at the medical school is a good starting point. The chief executive of a major university hospital can also be a productive source of options. Professional colleagues, regional and national medical associations, professional journal articles, and physician speakers at professional development meetings are also valuable sources.

Select at least three potential choices for a medical staff consultation. Ideally, a range of choices from a part-time consultant who is known as an expert in the particular challenge you face to a full-time consulting physician in a large firm would be optimal so that a clear choice is present. After identifying potential consultants, the next step is using a request for proposal (RFP) that articulates a clear objective and the scope of the engagement.

When analyzing the RFP responses, you should pay particular attention to the lead consultant and his or her approach to addressing the consulting engagement. A highly experienced consultant and a thoughtful work plan are necessities for a successful outcome.

Also, you should pay particular attention to reference checking for medical staff consultations. Often, these involve very delicate clinical quality or physician behavior challenges. Only the most skilled consultant will be able to maintain the level of respect needed to achieve positive outcomes. Communication skills are also essential in a medical staff consultant. Even the most brilliant consultant cannot be effective as a change agent unless he or she possesses strong communication abilities. Communication in this context means the ability to listen effectively, as well as to speak and write effectively.

Reference checks should help you determine if the medical staff consultant can be effective. In addition, the most promising consultants should receive personal interviews to assess his or her compatibility with the organization. Following personal interviews and after selecting the consultant, you're ready to begin the consultation.

PREREQUISITES FOR A SUCCESSFUL MEDICAL STAFF CONSULTATION

It takes a strong leader advocating the desired outcome to make a medical staff consultation successful. In the case of a quality improvement consultation for a medical staff, an elected chief of staff or a consensus of the department chairs is required for the desired improvement to succeed. In the case of a behavior modification consultation for an individual physician, it takes a respected colleague to insist upon change for the consultation to have a chance of success. For a financial consultation, it takes a dedicated executive leader to see the process of change through to a successful conclusion.

But a strong leader is not enough. The leader must advocate the "case" for the consultation and subsequent change. Virtually all medical staff consultations involve change, requiring an internal advocate to initiate the consulting process. Success also requires a consultant who can be an objective, creative, and motivated change agent. The consultant must be able to use the confidence and respect of physicians if he or she is to be effective.

Another prerequisite for a successful consultation is flexibility on the part of the organization leaders and a willingness to take an unpopular position when the situation calls for it. Consultation results are not always anticipated and the desired end result cannot be achieved unless a leader is able to adopt an uncompromising position.

Temper Tantrum Problem: The chief of staff of a community hospital faced what seemed to be an insurmountable problem. The vice president of nursing was pressing him to take disciplinary action against one of the most popular obstetricians in the hospital for constantly losing his temper and berating the nursing staff. The physician was admired by his patients, peers, and some of the nursing staff for his excellent clinical skills and patient relationships.

Other members of the nursing staff were extremely upset with his frequent losses of temper and loud outbursts, often in front of other employees and patients. After personally counseling the physician to no avail, the chief of staff turned to a consultant to assist him with resolving this delicate problem. The consultant listened patiently to physicians, staff, and even some patients who had been exposed to the temper tantrums. He also took care to interview the physician in question at great length. The consultant helped the chief of staff, vice president of nursing, and the nursing staff understand that the temper outbursts were usually the result of frustration with less than adequate nursing care, not unprovoked and meaningless attacks on individual nurses.

Once the core problems were identified, the nursing staff was able to achieve a higher level of skill through additional training, and the physician was able to modify his behavior and act as more of a teacher to the staff than an intimidator. The chief of staff credited the physician consultant with being an incredibly able and objective listener, two skills that assisted him in identifying and implementing a successful, although unforeseen, solution to the temper tantrums.

PITFALLS TO AVOID WITH MEDICAL STAFF CONSULTATIONS

The biggest pitfall to a medical staff consultation is failure to get started. Problems with a medical staff or an individual physician are by their nature delicate at best and emotionally charged at worst. Denial is a frequent response to medical staff or physician problems. It takes a committed leader to "call the question" when a serious but untreated problem exists. Retaining the right consultant can often make a very positive difference.

Another problem, not unique to medical staff consultations, is "bashing" the consultant if his or her analysis of the problem or the proposed solution is unpopular. Discrediting the consultant is a strategy sometimes employed when the real objective is to discredit the consultant's conclusions. Falling victim to this pitfall wastes precious time and money and rarely leads to an acceptable alternative solution.

Finally, becoming obsessed with the consulting project can also be a pitfall. Losing perspective during a consulting project can cause an entire organization to lose focus and can create problems greater than the consulting engagement was originally intended to change.

Too Much of a Good Thing: The president of a large medical clinic decided that the entire clinic organization needed a customer service overhaul. He observed that patients and families were rarely treated with the courtesy and respect he believed they deserved. He conducted a comprehensive search and retained a consulting firm that specialized in customer service improvement in medical clinics. He launched the engagement with much fanfare and promised to reinvent the clinic as a customer-driven organization.

The consulting engagement lasted over a year and required a seven-figure investment in professional fees. The clinic made great strides during the year in elevating its service standards and creating a revitalized customer-oriented culture. Employees at the clinic were highly enthusiastic, and the clinic president became a hero to them for championing the new culture. Physicians, however, were less enthusiastic.

Some physicians observed that all this "touchy-feely stuff" was taking money out of their pockets. At the end of the year, the clinic's profitability was reduced by the substantial consulting expenses and related investments in service improvements. The president was labeled as a "zealot" by his physician board and failed to win reelection. His successor discontinued the consultation and made it clear to the employees that, while good service was a goal, it was not to be an obsession in the future.

CHECKLIST FOR A SUCCESSFUL MEDICAL STAFF CONSULTATION

Initiating a medical staff consultation is a matter of good judgment. Rarely are there obvious signs of trouble that beg for a consultation. More often than not, subtle signs are the only indication that something is awry or an opportunity for change should be considered. Suggestions for a successful medical staff consultation include the following.

1. *Get started.* If you think there is a problem, act on it. Medical staff problems or problems with individual physicians rarely get better through neglect.
2. *Define the objective.* Before considering a consultation, you must define the desired outcome to be achieved.
3. *Select the best.* Find and retain the most capable consultant to help with the medical staff or physician issue. Retain the person with the best consulting credentials, not necessarily the person with the most impressive medical resume.
4. *Commit.* Be committed to listening to the consultant's advice and be prepared to follow it. If you did a good job hiring the consultant, trust his or her recommendations.

5. *Follow up.* Check back in a few months to be sure the implemented solution had the intended results. If it did not, make the necessary changes.

CONCLUSION

A clear opportunity exists to use more consultants in the medical staff area. These consultants may be harder to find than other types of consultants, but the search is well worth the effort. Thoughtfully deployed consultants working with effective organization leaders can achieve dramatic improvements in medical staff and individual physician performance.

Afterword: The Ideal Consultant

HIRING A CONSULTANT can help a healthcare organization solve an incredibly complicated problem or take full advantage of a defining moment of opportunity. It can also be a colossal waste of time and money leading to bitter disappointment. Selecting the best consultant, one that has all the ideal characteristics, makes the difference between success and failure. You should always seek the ideal consultant. Never settle for less.

The following six considerations are critical when searching for the ideal consultant.

1. *Honesty and integrity.* The ideal consultant always tells the truth. This is not always easy. A client may say he or she wants the truth, but not actually mean it; especially if the truth hurts. It is a rare consultant who can always tell a client the truth, especially if it is uncomfortable, inconvenient, or politically incorrect. Consultants who tell the truth run the risk of being fired if their clients are offended or defensive. Many consultants tell clients what they want to hear. The ideal consultant tells clients what they need to hear. He or she is not afraid of being fired or of resigning from a bad engagement if honesty and integrity are compromised. As a client, prepare yourself ahead of time to hear constructive criticism, or perhaps even unflattering observations, and commit to taking action.

2. *Client interests come first.* The ideal consultant always puts the client's interests first. The consultant's best resources are put into the engagement. Bait and switch tactics and upselling are never used. The ideal consultant always respects a client's confidentiality and never makes points at a client's expense.

3. *Experience.* The ideal consultant is experienced. At a minimum, the ideal consultant has at least three years experience working in the field of expertise he or she is consulting in and three or more years of experience as a consultant in that field. Clients should demand experienced consultants. The ideal consultant is not only experienced, but has a track record of helping clients achieve positive results. Consultants with limited experience are of limited value.

4. *Motivation.* The ideal consultant helps clients find their own way. Consultants do not tell clients how to do something—they simply help them discover the right method for their organization's best advantage. The ideal consultant is a teacher and a motivator. Anyone can give orders or instruct clients to do it "my way." The ideal consultant motivates and guides clients in finding their own way.

5. *Ability to say "No."* The ideal consultant can say "no" when it is appropriate. He or she can say no to a bad client when that client wants to do something fundamentally wrong or unethical, or say no to his or her own firm if the firm is going to do something counter to the best interests of his client. Saying no is an incredibly difficult task during demanding consulting engagements. Only the ideal consultant has the fortitude to do so.

6. *Communication skills.* The ideal consultant is a master of communication. He or she is skilled at listening, one of the lost arts of communication. The ideal consultant can communicate with clients in a manner that inspires rather than intimidates. The ideal consultant communicates just enough and never overwhelms the client. He or she maintains an open line of communication throughout and following a consulting engagement.

CONSULTANTS TO AVOID

If you can find a consultant with all or most of these six characteristics, you have found the ideal consultant. He or she will serve you and your organization extraordinarily well on any and every consulting engagement. But there are several types of consultants you should avoid.

Avoid the "face-man" consultant who shows up to sell the engagement but is not seen again until final report time. Avoid the "yes-man" consultant who tells clients what they want to hear and agrees with even the most inept ideas.

Avoid neophyte consultants with either little experience in consulting or the field in which they are providing advice. They have no place advising a good organization. Avoid mediocre consultants who have not had successful consulting outcomes in their field of expertise. Avoid "can't-do-teach" consultants who, after failing in their chosen profession, turn to consulting to make ends meet.

Avoid "company-man" consultants who are always looking to sell more work or advance their firm's interests over their clients' interests. Finally, avoid "Enron-man" consultants who, when faced with wrong-doing clients, write memos to cover themselves instead of taking action by forcing a change in their clients' behavior.

FINAL WORDS OF ADVICE

Use consultants only when absolutely necessary. Apply your organization's internal resources to solve problems and capitalize on opportunities whenever possible. If consultants are necessary, hire the very best, the ones closest to the ideal consultant. Listen to their advice. Combine consultants' wisdom with your own commitment and make positive changes.

Remember, extraordinary leadership achieves extraordinary results for your organization. Sometimes organizations can do it all themselves. At other times they need consulting help. Extraordinary leaders know the difference and act accordingly.

Appendix A

Sample Request for Proposal
Financial Performance Improvement

January 5, 2002

John A. Smith
Managing Partner
ABC Consolidated Consultants, LLC
100 Center Street
Anytown, Anystate 99999

Dear Mr. Smith,

Anytown General Hospital is considering retaining ABC Consolidated Consultants, LLC, to assist the hospital with improving its financial performance for the fiscal year 2003, beginning July 1, 2002. Your firm has been highly recommended by several of my professional colleagues, and I am most interested in receiving your response to this Request for Proposal.

I. ORGANIZATION AND PROPOSAL BACKGROUND
   A. *Organization Background:* Anytown General Hospital is a community-owned, nonprofit hospital that began operations in 1940. The hospital has a full range of acute care services and also operates two off-campus ambulatory surgery centers and one occupational medical center. At the present time, Anytown, a community of 250,000, has two other acute care hospitals. One is a for-profit hospital, and the second is a Catholic-sponsored facility that is part of a multi-state system.

Anytown General Hospital is governed by a fifteen-member Board of Trustees made up of community leaders. The hospital employs a total staff of 1,700 and has a medical staff of 300 physicians. Our annual operating budget is $205 million. The hospital has a seven-member administrative staff that consists of myself as president, one chief operating officer, and five vice presidents.

B. *Problem Background:* Anytown General Hospital has historically achieved a positive operating margin of 1 to 2 percent. For the most recent three fiscal years, our financial performance has deteriorated. The hospital projects an operating loss of 2 percent for the current fiscal year. The Board of Trustees and senior management have concluded that the hospital's financial performance must return to a positive 2 percent operating margin for the next fiscal year.

For the past two years senior management has tried various internal and consultant-assisted approaches to improve financial performance. Some improvements have been achieved; however, they have been short-lived and not sufficient to return the hospital to its historic levels of positive financial performance. Senior management has concluded that outside assistance is necessary to achieve our financial performance goals in fiscal year 2003.

C. *Objective of the Engagement:* The objective of this consultation is to assist senior management with developing all necessary plans to achieve a positive operating margin of 2 percent or greater in fiscal year 2003, which begins approximately six months from now.

D. *Scope, Timeframe, and Deliverables:* Anytown General Hospital desires to begin the consulting engagement no later than March 1, 2002, and conclude the engagement no later than June 30, 2002.

The desired scope of the engagement is as follows:

1. *Project Planning and Background Review*
   - Initial meetings with organization leaders
   - Review of pertinent background material
   - Planning meetings with senior management
2. *Financial Performance Improvement Initiatives*
   - Development of revenue improvement strategies

- Development of cost reduction strategies
- Completion of financial projections for FY 2003

3. *Management Structure Assessment*
   - Assessment of organization structures for overall hospital and all departments
   - Assessment of the strengths and weaknesses of senior administrative staff
   - Assessment of the strengths and weaknesses of all middle management staff

4. *Performance Improvement Plan Development*
   - Assist senior management with identifying sufficient revenue enhancement and cost reduction initiatives to achieve positive 2 percent operating margin in FY 2003
   - Prepare implementation schedule and plans to implement revenue and cost initiatives before beginning of FY 2003
   - Advise senior management on communication strategies for all key constituencies

5. *Report Preparation*
   - Preparation of draft report for review and approval by senior management
   - Oral presentation of report to Board of Trustees and senior management
   - Delivery of final written report

E. *Selection Criteria and Timeframe:* Anytown General Hospital is seeking proposals from five qualified consulting firms. The timeframe for our consultant selection is as follows:

January 5, 2002	Release request for proposals (RFPS)
January 31, 2002	RFP due to Anytown General Hospital
February 15, 2002	Selection of two finalist firms
March 1, 2002	Selection of consultant

Several consulting firms may be selected for site visits and interviews between January 31 and February 15, 2002. Two finalist firms will be interviewed between February 15 and March 1, 2002.

Anytown General Hospital will evaluate RFP responses, personal interview results, and professional references in order to make the final selection. Our key criteria will be qualifications of the firm and assigned consultants, approach to achieving our desired goals, professional fees, and quality of professional references. The specific expectations for RFP responses follow.

II. REQUEST FOR PROPOSAL EXPECTATIONS

    A. *Submission Expectations:* Five copies of your firm's completed proposal should be submitted by January 31, 2002, to:

        William F. Jones
        President and Chief Executive Officer
        Anytown General Hospital
        2100 State Street
        Anytown, Anystate 99999
        Phone: 999-999-9999

    B. *Proposal Format:* Proposals should follow this general format:

      1. *Qualifications of the Firm:* Describe your firm's history and general qualifications to perform healthcare organization financial performance improvement engagements.

      2. *Qualifications of the Consultants:* Describe the qualifications of the specific individual who will be the engagement leader and all of the staff consultants who will be active in the engagement. Specific emphasis should be placed on the qualifications of the engagement leader.

      3. *References:* Provide at least three, and preferably five, client references where your firm and the engagement leader have performed similar consulting assignments. The name, title, organization address, and contact phone number should be provided for each reference. It is preferable to have at least two references for organizations that worked with your firm 12 to 24 months ago to determine the long-term benefits of your financial performance improvement consultation.

      4. *Conflicts of Interest:* Describe any potential conflicts of interest that may be pertinent to this engagement.

      5. *Approach and Methodology:* Describe in detail the general approach and specific methodologies your firm will use to achieve the engagement objectives described above in Section I.D. In this section, you must also include a detailed

timetable to accommodate our desired start and completion dates as described in this RFP.

6. *Professional Fees and Expenses:* Specify the professional fees and all related expenses that are proposed to achieve this engagement. The desired payment schedule for professional fees must also be specified.

7. *Other Considerations:* Describe any other factors that might be relevant to our consideration of your firm's proposal. This is your opportunity to describe any unique strengths or capabilities that might influence our selection decision.

Thank you in advance for your interest in our engagement. Please feel free to contact me personally (999-999-9999) if you have any questions about the RFP or if our organization can supply you with any additional background material that may be useful in developing your proposal. I look forward to receiving your response on or before January 31, 2002.

Sincerely yours,

William F. Jones
President and Chief Executive Officer

Appendix B

Sample Letter of Engagement
Financial Performance Improvement

Professional Services Agreement Between Anytown General Hospital and ABC Consolidated Consultants, LLC

This Professional Services Agreement ("Agreement") is entered into as of the 1st day of March 2002 by and between Anytown General Hospital ("Hospital") and ABC Consolidated Consultants, LLC ("Company").

WHEREAS the Hospital desires to procure certain consultative professional services from the Company.

WHEREAS the Company desires to provide certain consultative professional services to the Hospital.

NOW THEREFORE, for and in consideration of the mutual covenants herein, the parties hereto agree as follows:

I. ENGAGEMENT OUTCOME
   The Company will work with senior management of the Hospital to develop a plan to achieve a 2 percent positive operating margin in fiscal year 2003.

II. SCOPE OF SERVICES
   The Company will assist Hospital senior management to identify financial performance improvement initiatives to achieve management's desired level of financial performance in FY 2003. Specifically, financial performance improvement opportunities in the areas of management, staff, supplies, clinical programs, and

service expenses will be evaluated. The approaches and timelines used to develop the strategic financial performance improvement plan for the Hospital are as follows:

A. *Project Planning and Background Material: April 1 to 19, 2002*
    1. Conduct initial meetings with members of the board, administrative staff, medical staff leaders, and middle management staff to introduce consultant and prepare the organization for the strategic financial performance improvement project.
    2. Project planning meetings with administrative staff to finalize overall financial performance improvement goal, project meeting schedules, and engagement methodology.
    3. Review pertinent financial background information to assist the Hospital during this engagement. Duplication of data already compiled during previous financial planning engagements will be avoided.
    4. Meet with other key advisors to the Hospital as requested by the President to coordinate the strategic financial performance improvement project.
    5. Review and evaluate recent consulting reports for revenue enhancement and cost reduction initiatives and integrate these initiatives as appropriate into future strategic financial performance improvement plans.

B. *Financial Performance Improvement Strategies: April 22 to June 7, 2002*
    1. Retreat (two to three hours) for administrative staff, medical staff leaders, and department managers to introduce consultant and initiate the strategic financial performance improvement project.
    2. Organize administrative staff and department managers into financial performance improvement task forces.
    3. Establish financial performance improvement goals for each task force.
    4. Implement review process and timetable for task force financial performance improvement recommendations.
    5. Hold board and medical staff education programs, as requested by the President, describing the need to implement financial performance improvement strategies in the future.

C. *Management Structure Review: May 6 to June 7, 2002*
  1. Review all departmental and administrative organization charts.
  2. Conduct individual meetings and focus groups with senior and middle management to evaluate management structure strengths and weaknesses.
  3. Review observations with the President and formulate organization structure improvements for future consideration.

D. *Draft Report Preparation: June 10 to 21, 2002*
  1. Review financial performance improvement recommendations with the President and senior management.
  2. Review management structure recommendations with the President and senior management.
  3. Prepare draft financial performance improvement plan and schedule of implementation.
  4. Hold management development retreat for senior management and department managers to review final financial performance improvement recommendations.

E. *Implementation Planning: June 17 to 28, 2002*
  1. Finalize staff and non-salary financial performance improvement implementation details.
  2. Conduct constituency communications, as requested by the President:
     - Board of Trustees
     - Management Staff
     - Medical Staff
  3. Present strategic financial performance improvement recommendations to President and Board of Trustees.
  4. Present final report to President and Board of Trustees.

III. PROFESSIONAL SERVICES

Consulting services will be provided by John A. Smith, Managing Partner; Mary Wilson, Senior Consultant; Janis Jones, Senior Consultant; and Lenore White, Staff Consultant. It is mutually agreed that John A. Smith will be the engagement leader for this engagement and will report directly to William F. Jones, President.

IV. TERM AND SCHEDULE

The term of this Agreement shall commence on March 1, 2002, and shall continue through June 30, 2002. The term of this Agreement may be amended by mutual agreement of the Company and the Hospital.

V. PROFESSIONAL FEES AND EXPENSES

The professional fees for this engagement are $350,000, payable as follows:

March 15, 2002	$50,000	Initial retainer
April 15, 2002	$50,000	Progress payment plus expenses
May 15, 2002	$100,000	Progress payment plus expenses
June 15, 2002	$100,000	Progress payment plus expenses
July 15, 2002	$50,000	Final payment plus expenses

The Company will provide detailed invoices for all out-of-pocket expenses for travel, accommodations, report preparation, etc., to the Hospital. All invoices will be provided to the Hospital 14 days in advance of due date. The Hospital agrees to pay Company's invoices on time.

VI. INDEMNIFICATION AND CONFIDENTIALITY

In engagements of this nature, it is the Company's practice to receive indemnification. Accordingly, in consideration of our agreement to act on your behalf in connection with this assignment, the Hospital agrees to indemnify and hold the Company, and any affiliated companies, harmless from any and all losses, claims, damages, or liabilities incurred by them or to which they may become subject in connection to this engagement.

The Hospital agrees to reimburse the Company and any other person indemnified hereunder for any legal or other expenses, including professional time, as they are reasonably incurred in connection with investigating or defending any such loss, claim, damage, or liability.

Information in this engagement letter proposal is confidential and proprietary to the Company. No information contained in this engagement letter proposal may be disclosed to any party outside of the Hospital without the written approval in advance of the Company.

The Company acknowledges that in working with the Hospital they may be provided confidential information and may participate in meetings of a confidential nature. The Company agrees not to disclose any confidential information about the Hospital to any other party.

VII. MISCELLANEOUS

A. *Notices:* Any notice or other communication required or permitted hereunder shall be in writing and shall, unless personally delivered into the hands of the party to be notified or the proper agents of that party, be deemed effectively given as of the date of mailing thereof by certified mail, with postage and certification fees prepaid, to the party to be notified.

B. *Governing Law:* The parties agree that this Agreement shall be construed and governed in accordance with the laws of Anystate.

C. *Entire Agreement:* This Agreement constitutes the entire Agreement between the parties and contains all of the Agreements between the parties with respect to the subject matter hereof; this Agreement supersedes any and all other Agreements, either oral or in writing, between the parties hereto with respect to the subject matter hereof.

D. *Amendments:* No amendment or modification of this Agreement shall be valid or binding on either party unless made in writing and signed by a duly authorized agent of both parties. No waiver of any provision of this Agreement shall be valid unless in writing and signed by the person or party to be charged.

E. *Enforceability:* If any portion or portions of this Agreement shall be, for any reason, held to be invalid or unenforceable, the remaining portion or portions shall nevertheless be valid, enforceable and carried into effect.

F. *Text Controls:* Section headings and numbers have been inserted herein for convenience of reference only, and if there shall be any conflict between such numbers or headings and the text of the Agreement, the text shall control.

G. *Assignment:* The Company may not assign this Agreement or any part of this Agreement to any successor or third party.

VIII. SIGNATURES OF THE PARTIES

IN WITNESS OF THE FOREGOING the Hospital and the Company have caused this Agreement to be duly executed on the 1st day of March 2002.

ANYTOWN GENERAL HOSPITAL   ABC CONSOLIDATED COMPANY, LLC
("Hospital")   ("Company")

By:_____   By:_____
President and Chief   Managing Partner
Executive Officer

Appendix C

Sample Request for Proposal Governance Performance Improvement

January 5, 2003

Richard A. Beneficial, President
Beneficial Associates, Inc.
100 Center Street
Ourtown, Ourstate 88888

Dear Mr. Beneficial,

Twin Peaks Regional Medical Center is considering retaining Beneficial Associates, Inc., to assist our organization with evaluating the performance of the Board of Directors and preparing an action plan to make improvements in the Board's performance. Your firm has been highly recommended by several of my professional colleagues, and I am most interested in having you respond to this Request for Proposal.

I. ORGANIZATION AND PROPOSAL BACKGROUND

A. *Organization Background:* Twin Peaks Regional Medical Center is a community-owned, not-for-profit medical center that began operations in 1995 following the merger of Twin Peaks General Hospital and Twin Peaks Medical Clinics. Both of the organizations had been in operation since the 1930s preceding the merger.

Twin Peaks is a community of 65,000 residents. There are no other hospitals in the immediate area, but several large and sophisticated medical centers are located within a 30-minute drive.

The Medical Center has an annual operating budget of $115 million. Our organization employees a staff of 1,250 and has a total medical staff of 200, of which 50 are employed by the Medical Center.

Twin Peaks Regional Medical Center is governed by a Board of Directors consisting of 24 members. Twelve of the Directors were selected from the Twin Peaks General Hospital Board and 12 were selected from the Twin Peaks Medical Center Board at the time of the merger.

B. *Problem Background:* The Board of Directors for Twin Peaks Regional Medical Center has concluded that the governing Board is not performing its duties effectively. The Board experiences frequent deadlocks on key issues with Directors voting along their pre-merger affiliation lines. The Board has not coalesced into an effective governance team following the merger of 1995.

During past annual retreats, Directors have expressed their enthusiasm for making improvements in the governance process, but no sustained changes have occurred. The Medical Center has experienced turnover of three chief executives since the merger occurred eight years ago. I have recently begun my tenure as the organization's fourth chief executive. I have a strong desire to work with my Board early in my tenure to improve governance effectiveness so that the Board and administration can become an effective leadership team.

C. *Objective of the Engagement:* Twin Peaks Regional Medical Center desires to conduct a comprehensive governance performance improvement consultation consisting of the following:
1. Assessing current governance weaknesses
2. Identifying performance improvement initiatives
3. Deliberating alternative governance improvement strategies
4. Gaining consensus on desired improvements
5. Developing an implementation action plan

It is our desire as an organization to significantly improve governance performance to support the overall success and growth of Twin Peaks Regional Medical Center.

D. *Scope, Timeframe, and Deliverables:* Twin Peaks Regional Medical Center desires to begin the consulting engagement April 1, 2003, and conclude the engagement no later than October 31, 2003.

The desired scope of the engagement is as follows:

1. *Assessing Current Weaknesses:* The governing Board desires to evaluate its performance in all aspects of governance and implement strategies to improve its performance and set a positive example for the organization as a whole. At a minimum, the following aspects shall be carefully evaluated:
   - Board organization and committees
   - Director selection and orientation
   - Director job description and performance expectations
   - Conflict of interest expectations
   - Continuing education and officer succession planning
   - Confidentiality requirements
   - Governance policies

2. *Identifying Performance Improvement Initiatives:* The consultant will review governance policies, minutes of governing Board and committee meetings for the previous 12 months, and all internal and external reports relevant to the performance of the Board (e.g., JCAHO accreditation reports, financial audit, strategic plan). The consultant will attend, as guest observer, two Board meetings and four committee meetings to gain firsthand knowledge of the Board in action. In addition, the consultant will interview all Board members, senior management, and medical staff leaders to gain their insights.

3. *Deliberating Alternative Governance Improvement Strategies:* Based on the review of background material, attendance at key meetings, and personal interviews, the consultant will assess the Board's strengths and weaknesses, provide several initial ideas for performance improvement, and develop preliminary recommendations that will be presented to the Board for further refinement and discussion.

4. *Gaining Consensus on Desired Improvements:* The consultant will facilitate further discussion among the Board members to build consensus on the desired initiatives for governance performance improvement. Although unanimity may not be achievable, consensus is absolutely critical.

5. *Developing an Implementation Action Plan:* In conjunction with the chief executive and Board leaders, the consultant will prepare an action plan that identifies specific initiatives, a defined timeframe, and follow-up actions to implement the desired governance performance improvements.

6. *Selection Criteria and Timeframe:* Twin Peaks Regional Medical Center is seeking proposals from five qualified consulting firms. The timeframe for consultant selection is as follows:

January 5, 2003	Release request for proposals (RFPS)
January 31, 2003	RFPS due at Twin Peaks Regional Medical Center
February 28, 2003	Selection of two finalist firms
March 31, 2003	Selection of consultant

At least two finalist firms will be selected for interviews in March 2003 based on the quality of the RFPS submitted. Our key criteria for selecting finalists and making the selection of the consultant will be the qualifications, references, and personal interview results of the engagement leader. Of course, professional fees will also be a consideration in our selection process. The specific expectations for the RFP responses are as follows:

II. REQUEST FOR PROPOSAL EXPECTATIONS

A. *Submission Expectations:* Five copies of your firm's completed proposal should be submitted to:

Malcolm F. Middle
President and Chief Executive Officer
Twin Peaks Regional Medical Center
Twin Peaks, Anystate 99999
Phone: 999-999-9999

B. *Proposal Format:* Proposals should follow this general format:
  1. *Qualifications of the Firm:* Describe your firm's history and general qualifications to perform governance performance improvement engagements.
  2. *Qualifications of the Consultants:* Describe the qualifications of the specific individual who will be the engagement leader and all of the staff consultants who will be active in the engagement. Specific emphasis should be placed on the qualifications of the engagement leader.

     Please provide at least three, and preferably five, client references where your firm and the engagement leader have performed similar consulting assignments. The name, title, organization address, and contact phone number should be provided for each reference. It is preferable to have at least two references for organizations that worked with your firm 12 to 24 months ago to determine the long-term benefits of your governance consultation.

     Finally, please describe any potential conflicts of interest that may be pertinent to this engagement.
  3. *Approach and Methodology:* Describe in detail the general approach and specific methodologies your firm will use to achieve the engagement deliverables described in Section 1.D. In this section, you must also include a detailed timetable to accommodate our desired start and completion dates, described earlier in this RFP.
  4. *Professional Fees and Expenses:* Specify the professional fees and all related expenses that are proposed to achieve this engagement. The desired payment schedule for professional fees must also be specified.
  5. *Other Considerations:* Describe any other factors that might be relevant to our consideration of your firm's proposal. This is your opportunity to describe any unique strengths or capabilities that might influence our selection decision.

Thank you in advance for your interest in our engagement. Please feel free to contact me personally (999-999-9999) if you have any questions about the RFP or if our organization can supply you with any additional background material that may be useful in developing your proposal. I look forward to receiving your response on or before January 31, 2003.

Sincerely yours,

Malcolm F. Middle
President and Chief Executive Officer

cc: Gerald Q. Jones
        Chairman, Board of Directors

Appendix D

*Sample Governance Policy Manual
Table of Contents and Sample Policies*

BOARD OF TRUSTEES POLICY MANUAL
ANYTOWN GENERAL HOSPITAL

TABLE OF CONTENTS

		Page
PREAMBLE		iii
1.	GOVERNING BOARD POLICIES	
1A	Board of Trustees Mission Statement	1
1B	Governing Board Organization and Committees	3
1C	Governing Board Meetings	6
1D	Trustee Qualifications and Selection	9
1E	Trustee Orientation	13
1F	Trustee Responsibilities	16
1G	Trustee Performance Standards and Reappointment	20
1H	Governing Board Evaluation	23
1I	Trustee Continuing Education	25
1J	Trustee Succession Planning	27
1K	Trustee Conflict of Interest	29
1L	Trustee Compensation and Reimbursement	33
1M	Trustee Confidentiality	35
1N	Governing Board Bylaws	36
1O	Accreditation and JCAHO Standards	38

1P	Performance Improvement	39
1Q	Advisors to the Board	41

2. COMMUNICATION POLICIES

2A	Board of Trustees Communication	43
2B	Medical Staff Communication	45
2C	Leader and Partner Communication	47
2D	Community Relations	49
2E	Complaint Follow-up and Resolution	51

3. HOSPITAL PRESIDENT POLICIES

3A	Hospital President Recruitment and Selection	52
3B	Hospital President Position Description	55
3C	Hospital President Evaluation and Compensation	61
3D	Senior Management Development and Succession Planning	65
3E	Senior Management Incentive Compensation	67
3F	Key Management Extra-hospital Activities	70

4. FINANCE AND PLANNING POLICIES

4A	Annual Operating Plan	72
4B	Financial Authority Limits	75
4C	Strategic Planning	78
4D	Investment Planning	80
4E	Anytown General Hospital Foundation	82

APPENDIX A. BOARD OF TRUSTEES SELF-EVALUATION SURVEY A1	85

ANYTOWN GENERAL HOSPITAL
BOARD OF TRUSTEES POLICY MANUAL
GOVERNING BOARD POLICIES

Subject: Trustee Performance Standards and Reappointment
Approval Date: February 2001
Number: 1G

I. POLICY

Trustees of Anytown General Hospital are responsible for fulfilling the Trustee responsibilities and duties described in Policy 1F. Performance on these general and specific duties contributes to the Board's overall effectiveness and the Hospital's success in fulfilling its mission. It is the policy of the Board to base reappointment to the Board on willingness to serve and perform in accordance with the following Trustee performance standards.

II. IMPLEMENTATION

To contribute to the excellent performance of the Board as a whole, Trustees are expected to fulfill the following standards:

A. *Performance Standards*
   1. Prepare for Board and committee meetings through the study and preparatory work necessary for intelligent discussion.
   2. Attend meetings of the Board and assigned committees.
   3. Perform Board assignments promptly.
   4. Maintain confidentiality and security regarding Hospital information.
   5. Contribute positively to Board discussions, assisting the Board in reaching conclusions.
   6. Serve as a consultant and advisor to the Hospital President and, with his or her approval, to others in the organization.
   7. Acquire a working knowledge of those functional activities for which he or she has committee assignments.
   8. Develop a broad knowledge of current and future trends in healthcare.
   9. Be alert to new program opportunities and assist the organization on specific programs when requested.
   10. Avoid interfering or the appearance of interfering in Hospital operations.

11. Avoid conflicts of interest or the appearance of conflicts of interest. Trustees or their professional affiliates may not accept any paid work from Anytown General Hospital.

12. Maintain a positive attitude toward the Board, medical staff, and administration at all times with external parties and the community.

13. Review Hospital performance against mission and goals and take corrective action when mission or goals are not being achieved.

14. Adhere to the highest standards of integrity and ethics and avoid any actions which are or appear to be inconsistent with such standards.

B. *Reappointment*

The Executive Committee of the Board of Trustees reviews Trustees for reappointment at the end of each Trustee's term. This review will include, but not be limited to the following:

1. Trustee's demonstrated interest in service on the Board as shown by:
   - attendance;
   - active participation in meetings; and
   - affirmation that he or she desires to be reappointed.

2. Participation in continuing education programs.

3. Potential conflicts of interest.

4. Collaborative relationships with other Trustees.

5. Health status.

6. Ability to commit required time to the anticipated future demands of Board membership.

7. Active support for the Board of Trustees, administration, and medical staff of Anytown General Hospital.

C. *Removal*

All Trustees are expected to fulfill their responsibilities as Trustees in accordance with the Trustee Performance Standards. Failure to perform shall be grounds for removal from the Board of Trustees.

III. RESPONSIBILITY

The responsibility for fulfilling the duties of Trustees rests with each Trustee and is periodically reviewed by the Chairperson of the Board.

ANYTOWN GENERAL HOSPITAL
BOARD OF TRUSTEES POLICY MANUAL
GOVERNING BOARD POLICIES

Subject: Advisors to the Board
Approval Date: February 2001
Number: 1Q

I. POLICY
    It is the policy of the Board that independent advisors should be
    retained periodically to evaluate the Hospital's financial, quality,
    and governance performance.

II. IMPLEMENTATION
    A. *Financial Audit*
        The Fiscal Management and Audit Committee of the Board,
        subject to the approval of the Board, engages an independent
        Certified Public Accounting firm to conduct the annual review
        of the financial position for the Hospital and any other financial
        reviews desired by the committee. The Fiscal Management and
        Audit Committee will periodically (at least every five years)
        evaluate the performance of the Certified Public Accounting
        firm and may, at its discretion, obtain competitive proposals
        from alternate firms.
    B. *Legal Advisors*
        The Executive Committee of the Board, in consultation with the
        Hospital President, engages a qualified law firm to handle gen-
        eral legal and corporate matters for the Hospital. The law firm
        will prepare an annual report for the Board on all matters of
        importance, as determined by the Executive Committee and
        Board of Trustees Compliance Committee. The Hospital
        President will periodically (at least every five years) evaluate the
        performance of the law firm and may, at his or her discretion,
        obtain competitive proposals from alternate firms.
    C. *Governance Audit*
        The Chairperson of the Board, in conjunction with the Executive
        Committee, will periodically (at least every five years) appoint a
        governance advisor to conduct an independent review of the

Board's performance and develop recommendations for improvement of the governance process.

D. *Quality of Care*

The Executive Committee, in conjunction with the Hospital President, may retain independent medical advisors to evaluate the quality of medical services provided by the Hospital. The reviews will be conducted any time the Board, administration or medical staff leadership desires to obtain an independent assessment of a Hospital service or an individual medical staff member. The results of any quality of care review will be communicated to the Board of Trustees.

E. *Other Advisors*

The Board may appoint other independent advisors from time to time to conduct special reviews. Examples of such reviews include:

- Internal controls
- Strategic affiliations
- Investment performance

III. IMPLEMENTATION

The responsibility for overseeing the Advisors to the Board Policy is assigned to the Chairperson of the Board and the Executive Committee of the Board.

ANYTOWN GENERAL HOSPITAL
BOARD OF TRUSTEES POLICY MANUAL
COMMUNICATION POLICIES

Subject: Board of Trustees Communication
Approval Date: February 2001
Number: 2A

I. POLICY

The Board of Trustees is committed to receiving full and honest communication from the Hospital President about the current and future state of the Hospital. It is the policy of the Board that the Hospital President fully communicate both positive and negative aspects of the Hospital's operation so that appropriate action can be taken by the Board to ensure the Hospital fulfills its mission.

II. IMPLEMENTATION

A. *Monthly Board Report*

The Hospital President will prepare a monthly Operations Report for the Board that summarizes the key aspects of the Hospital's operations for the previous month. This report shall be submitted monthly, regardless of whether or not a Board meeting is scheduled. The monthly Operations Report shall contain discussion of current and projected problems as well as the Hospital President's plans to address problems.

B. *Dashboard Reports*

The Hospital President shall from time to time prepare a "dashboard" report for Trustees which highlights operational, financial, and clinical indicators in a highly condensed format. This report will be used during times of fiscal distress and at other such times as requested by the Board.

C. *Board Meetings*

The Hospital President shall deliver an oral report to the Board of Trustees at all scheduled meetings and committee meetings. The Hospital President's report shall be candid and contain both positive and negative aspects of the Hospital's performance.

D. *Trustee Meetings*

The Hospital President shall meet individually with all Trustees at least annually to solicit Trustee input and to receive Trustee counsel. The Hospital President and Trustees are mutually expected to be thorough and candid in all discussions with each other.

III. RESPONSIBILITY

Responsibility for implementing the Board of Trustees Communication Policy is assigned to the Chairperson of the Board.

ANYTOWN GENERAL HOSPITAL
BOARD OF TRUSTEES POLICY MANUAL
HOSPITAL PRESIDENT POLICIES

Subject: Hospital President Recruitment and Selection
Approval Date: February 2001
Number: 3A

I. POLICY

The recruitment and selection of the Hospital President is one of the most important functions of the Anytown General Hospital Board of Trustees. It is the policy of the Board to organize an ad hoc President's Search Committee for the purpose of hiring the best candidate available to lead Anytown General Hospital when a vacancy occurs in the Office of the President.

II. IMPLEMENTATION

A. *President's Search Committee*

The Chairperson of the Board will designate individuals for a President's Search Committee using following guidelines:

1. The Chairperson of the Board, previous Chairpersons, and other interested and qualified Trustees may be members of the committee. Trustees who have had prior experience with executive selection in their own organizations, for example, would be appropriate. The President of the Medical Staff will also serve on the committee.
2. The Search Committee shall have sufficient members so that varied viewpoints of the Board are represented.
3. The Search Committee chairperson shall be selected for his or her leadership ability and ability to get things done in a climate of mutual respect.
4. The Search Committee will be charged specifically with finding and evaluating candidates and making a recommendation for approval of a finalist to the full Board.
5. The Search Committee may retain an executive search consultant who specializes in the healthcare field if it is deemed necessary.
6. The Search Committee, in conjunction with the Board of Trustees, will delineate the desired personal and professional

characteristics of persons likely to be acceptable to the committee. The Search Committee will establish a reasonable schedule for finding, screening and investigating potential candidates and will report on the progress at least monthly to the full Board. The Search Committee will meet as necessary and communicate regularly with the search consultant, if retained, to provide necessary information and data for candidates.

7. The Search Committee will conduct formal interviews of candidates deemed to meet the Hospital's search criteria.

B. *Final Candidate Selection*

After the Search Committee has evaluated initial candidates and identified two or three final candidates, references should be thoroughly checked by committee members and the search consultant. The Search Committee should then make its selection recommendation of the top candidate after a second interview and interviews with administrative staff and the Medical Staff Executive Committee. Upon completion of the interviews, the search process should be finalized as follows:

1. The final position description and Board expectations should be defined.

2. The candidate's salary and benefit expectations should be identified.

3. An optional site visit to the finalist candidate's current facility may be made by two or three members of the Search Committee.

4. The formal job offer should be formulated and communicated by telephone to the candidate by the Chairperson of the Board.

5. Upon oral acceptance, a written letter of agreement should be drafted and executed by the Executive Committee.

6. Upon receipt of the signed letter of agreement, an appropriate announcement to the Hospital and medical staff should be released by the Chairperson of the Board. Additionally, suitable public announcements should be released to the local media.

7. Thank you letters to all candidates should be sent following completion of the Hospital President search.

C. *Hospital President's Arrival*

When the new Hospital President arrives, the Board of Trustees will host a reception to welcome him or her to Anytown General Hospital and the community. Those invited should include: Trustees, medical staff, Hospital leaders, and community leaders.

III. RESPONSIBILITY

Responsibility for the Hospital President Recruitment and Selection Policy will be assigned to an ad hoc President's Search Committee, appointed by the Board, and the Chairperson of the Board.

ANYTOWN GENERAL HOSPITAL
BOARD OF TRUSTEES POLICY MANUAL
FINANCE AND PLANNING POLICIES

Subject: Financial Authority Limits
Approval Date: February 2001
Number: 4B

I. POLICY

Anytown General Hospital acknowledges that the Hospital President is responsible for administering the day-to-day operation of the Hospital. To carry out these responsibilities effectively, the Board of Trustees delegates certain authorities to the Hospital President and the Hospital President is expected to function within the authority limits designated by this policy.

II. IMPLEMENTATION

A. *Capital Equipment*

The Hospital President is authorized to purchase all items of capital equipment, after approval of the annual capital plan. The Hospital President may purchase items not in the approved capital budget of up to $100,000 if appropriate eliminations are made in approved items so that the overall approved capital budget is not exceeded.

Leases approved in the annual capital plan of up to $100,000 for the life of the lease may be approved by the Hospital President. All leases valued at more than $100,000 require the approval of the Board.

B. *Management Staff Salaries*

The Hospital President is authorized to perform annual evaluations and grant salary increases to all members of the management staff. The Hospital President will present an overall percentage and dollar budget for management salary increases to the Board as part of the annual financial plan. On approval of the annual financial plan, the Hospital President is authorized to grant raises throughout the year consistent with management performance and the approved budget.

C. *Employee Compensation*

The Hospital President is authorized to implement pay increases for all Hospital employees. The Hospital President will present an overall percentage and dollar budget for employee salary increases to the Board as part of the annual financial plan. On approval of the annual financial plan, the Hospital President is authorized to grant raises throughout the year consistent with employee performance and market conditions.

D. *Professional Contracts*

The Hospital President is authorized to negotiate and sign professional service contracts for physicians, consultants, architects and so forth, for up to $100,000. The President is expected to ensure that professional service contracts are in compliance with all pertinent regulatory requirements. The Hospital President will present an overall dollar budget for professional services as part of the annual financial plan. On approval of the plan, the Hospital President is authorized to enter into professional service contracts necessary to further the interests of Anytown General Hospital.

E. *Legal Settlements*

The Hospital President is authorized to settle lawsuits or potential lawsuits against the Hospital for up to $100,000 per occurrence, upon consultation with the Hospital's legal counsel. Settlements greater than $100,000 must be approved by the Board of Trustees Executive Committee.

F. *Litigation Opportunities*

The Hospital President is authorized to proceed or forego litigation opportunities in the amount of $100,000 or less. Proceeding with or foregoing litigation opportunities above $100,000 must be approved by the Board of Trustees Executive Committee.

G. *Purchase or Sale of Property*

The Hospital President is authorized to sell used Hospital equipment valued at $100,000 or less in the course of normal operations of the Hospital. The Hospital President is not authorized to purchase or to sell real estate property or buildings without approval by the Board of Trustees.

III. RESPONSIBILITY

The Hospital's independent auditor is assigned the responsibility to determine whether or not the Hospital President has functioned within the Financial Authority Limits Policy.

These authority limits will be reviewed biennially by the Fiscal Management and Audit Committee and changed as necessary.

Appendix E

Sample Request for Proposal Audit Services

December 3, 2002

Herbert S. Smith, Partner
A-One Accounting
1400 Lake Boulevard, Suite 400
Anytown, Anystate 99999

Dear Mr. Smith,

St. Mary Hospital ("SMH") is in the process of selecting an accounting firm to perform annual audit services for fiscal year 2004 and subsequent years. The annual audit is to include SMH and related enterprises. SMH is interested in retaining an accounting firm experienced with providing audit services to Catholic health systems and hospitals. SMH submits this Request for Proposal (RFP) to provide an opportunity for your firm to present a proposal for these services.

I. BACKGROUND

SMH is a Catholic hospital sponsored by the Sisters of Holiness. SMH is a tax-exempt Ourstate not-for-profit corporation that provides acute hospital care and other related healthcare services to residents on the southwest side of Ourtown. SMH recently has undertaken a reorganization of its Board of Trustees and administrative leadership. SMH appointed a new chief executive officer and a new chief financial officer in 2002. The Board of Trustees and senior management desire to select a new accounting firm to provide audit services beginning with the fiscal year 2004 audit for the period ending June 30, 2004. SMH has experienced a period of disappointing financial performance for fiscal years 1999–2003, but is making significant progress in improving performance in 2003.

II. PROPOSAL OBJECTIVES

SMH will select a new accounting firm that is able to accomplish the following:

A. Demonstrate the ability of the firm to provide high quality audit services;

B. Demonstrate the ability to assign the most capable and professional partner and support staff;

C. Provide constructive and candid advice and counsel to the Board of Trustees, chief executive officer, and chief financial officer; and

D. Propose creative and collaborative "value" billing methodologies that will reduce annual audit fees by 20 to 30 percent in 2004 and subsequent years.

III. RFP EVALUATION CRITERIA

Your proposal will be evaluated to determine the degree to which it is responsive to the requirements of SMH. The following criteria will be used to evaluate the proposals:

A. Quality of the proposal and responsiveness to the RFP requirements and the firm's ability to represent SMH in a high-quality and cost-effective manner

B. Overall qualifications, experience, and track record of the firm to provide audit services

C. Specific qualifications and experience of the audit partner to be assigned to SMH

D. The firm's ability to provide pro-active and candid advice to the Board and senior management leaders

IV. PROPOSAL REQUIREMENTS

Please respond to the following questions in a clear and thorough manner:

A. *Firm Experience and Background*
   - Describe in a concise manner the history of your firm and its strengths. Include a profile of your firm and description of

its composition, significant areas of practice, and number of partners and support staff.

- Attach resumes of all key personnel who will handle the SMH audit if your firm is selected. Clearly identify the partner who will be responsible for SMH activity.
- Provide references for five hospitals for which your firm has provided audit services. Ideally, references should be for Catholic-sponsored hospitals of similar size, market area, and payer mix. Also provide an individual reference to contact at each institution, including address and phone number of the contact.

B. *Conflict of Interest*
- Identify any actual or potential conflict of interest, which would affect your selection as auditors for SMH.

C. *Fee Structure*
- Describe the usual and customary billing arrangements for individuals your firm anticipates assigning to SMH.
- Please propose an innovative fee arrangement designed to reduce SMH's audit expense by 20 to 30 percent in future years.

D. *Other Information*
- Provide any other pertinent information that would assist SMH in evaluating your firm's qualifications to serve as SMH's auditor.

V. SCOPE OF SERVICES EXPECTATIONS

SMH expects its audit firm to meet the following expectations:

A. *Audit*

Provision of annual audit services for SMH consistent with current generally accepted accounting standards.

B. *Audit Timeframe*

Timeframe expectations for completing audit are:
- Draft Audit for senior management review: mid-August.
- Completed audit for Board Finance Committee review: mid-September.
- Completed audit for board review: late September.

C. *Value-Added Services*
- SMH's audit firm will be expected to provide at least one Board Finance Committee education program per year. Topic to be selected by SMH.
- SMH's audit firm will be expected to provide a mid-year progress report to the Finance Committee and full board of Trustees in March of each year highlighting management's progress in addressing Management Letter issues or any other outstanding financial issues from the previous year's audit.

D. *Reporting Expectations*

SMH's audit firm is expected to report directly to the Chairman, Board of Trustees Finance Committee. The audit firm selected will work closely with the chief executive officer, chief financial officer, and members of the Finance Department staff.

E. *Integrity Expectations*

SMH's audit firm will be expected to be thoroughly candid and objective in all oral and written communications with SMH and its Board and senior management representatives.

VI. PROPOSAL SUBMISSION

In order to consider your proposal, a timely response to this request in the form of one original signed proposal and four copies must be received no later than December 28, 2002. Please send your proposal to

Edward X. White
Vice President and Chief Financial Officer
St. Mary Hospital
400 Elm Avenue
Ourtown, Ourstate 88888

SMH will evaluate RFP responses and interview at least two finalist firms in January 2003. It is our intent to select our new auditor no later than March 1, 2003.

VII. PROPOSAL PREPARATION

If you need any clarification or have any questions, you may contact me at 999-999-9999. Background noted on the hospital and previous audits will be made available at your request. After reviewing your proposal, it is possible that SMH may want to interview representatives of your firm. SMH's objective is to review proposals in January 2003, interview selected firms in February, and appoint our new audit firm by March 1, 2003.

Thank you in advance for your interest. We look forward to receiving your response.

Sincerely yours,

Edward X. White
Vice President and Chief Financial Officer

Appendix F

Sample Request for Proposal
Legal Services

March 29, 2003

John Doe, Esq.
Lead Healthcare Partner
Able, Baker, and Charlie LLC
100 Center Street
Ourtown, Ourstate 88888

Dear Mr. Doe,

Saint Mary Hospital ("SMH") is in the process of selecting a law firm to serve as the hospital's primary provider of legal services. SMH is interested in developing a preferred legal services provider arrangement with a law firm in the areas of general corporate healthcare and related transactions, including, but not limited to: anti-trust, tax, corporate, employee benefits, intellectual property, labor/employment, medical staff, patient care, reimbursement, and regulatory matters. SMH is also interested in retaining a firm with experience serving Catholic healthcare systems and hospitals. SMH submits this Request for Proposal (RFP) to provide an opportunity for your firm to present a proposal for these services.

I. BACKGROUND

SMH is a Catholic hospital sponsored by the Sisters of Holiness. SMH is a tax-exempt Ourstate not-for-profit corporation that provides acute hospital care and other related healthcare services. For your information, we are enclosing an overview of the SMH organization. SMH currently spends approximately $500,000 annually on legal services. sMH recently has undertaken a reorganization of its Board of Trustees and administrative leadership. The Board and new President desire to select a new law firm to advise the Hospital on legal matters in the future.

II. PROPOSAL OBJECTIVES
sMH will select a new law firm that is able to accomplish the following:
A. Demonstrate the ability of the firm to provide high quality legal representation
B. Demonstrate immediate access to address urgent problems
C. Provide legal representation in a cost-effective manner
D. Propose creative and collaborative "value" billing mechanisms for legal representation that will reduce overall legal expenses by 20 to 30 percent or greater in future years.

III. RFP EVALUATION CRITERIA
Your proposal will be evaluated to determine the degree to which it is responsive to the requirements of sMH. The following criteria will be used to evaluate the proposals:
A. Quality of the proposal and responsiveness to the RFP requirements, and the firm's ability to represent sMH in a high-quality and cost-effective manner
B. Overall qualifications, experience, client service and/or representation philosophy of the firm; commitment of the firm to provide the services, expertise, and staff as set forth in the proposal
C. Qualifications and experience of the lead counsel assigned to sMH
D. The firm's creativity and flexibility in determining the appropriate legal services provided, as well as the appropriate compensation/fee structure to provide the requested services
E. Firm's experience in the various areas of law required by sMH
F. Firm's ability to provide proactive consulting advice to the Board and administration

IV. PROPOSAL REQUIREMENTS
Please respond to the following questions in a clear and thorough manner:

A. *Firm Experience and Background*
- Describe in a clear and concise manner the history of your firm including its strengths and significant practice areas. Please include a profile of your firm including a summary of the number of partners and associates.
- Attach resumes of all principal attorneys who will handle SMH matters and other select members of your firm whom you propose to have assist in representing SMH. Attorney resumes should clearly describe corporate, healthcare, and transactional experience. Also identify the specific attorney who will be designated lead counsel to SMH.
- Provide three references of healthcare institutions for which your law firm has acted as lead counsel. Describe any innovative or creative elements of these client arrangements. Also provide an individual to contact at each institution, including address and phone number of the contact.

B. *Conflict of Interest*
Identify any actual or potential conflict of interest which would affect your representation of SMH.

C. *Fee Structure*
- Describe the usual and customary billing arrangements for individuals your firm anticipates assigning to SMH.
- Please propose innovative fee arrangements that are designed to promote a preferred legal services provider arrangement between your firm and SMH. Describe your overall approach to working with SMH's leadership to reduce legal fees by 20 to 30 percent in future years.

D. Other Information
Please provide any other pertinent information that would assist us in evaluating your firm's qualifications to serve as SMH's lead counsel.

V. PROPOSAL SUBMISSION
In order to consider your proposal, a timely response to this request in the form of one original signed proposal and six copies must be received no later than April 20, 2003. Please send your proposal to:

Charles E. Brown, President
St. Mary Hospital
400 Elm Avenue
Ourtown, Ourstate 88888

VI. PROPOSAL PREPARATION

If you need any clarification or have any questions, you may contact me at 999-999-9999. After reviewing your proposal to serve as SMH's preferred provider for legal services, it is possible that we will want to interview representatives of your firm. If selected for interview, your firm will be expected to make a brief presentation summarizing your proposal and respond to questions. SMH's objective is to select our new legal provider and transition our legal work to the firm selected in May 2003.

Thank you in advance for your interest. We look forward to your response.

Sincerely yours,

Charles E. Brown
President

Appendix G

Sample Letter of Engagement Human Resources Consultation

August 15, 2003

William F. Gardner, M.D.
President and Chief Executive Officer
Four Plants Medical Clinics
100 State Street
Botanical Grove, Anystate 33333

Dear Dr. Gardner,

Human Resource Insights, LLC, is pleased to provide Four Plants Medical Clinics with consulting services relative to the evaluation of your Human Resources Department and development of an action plan to improve the department's operation. Given the organization's recent trends of high employee turnover, increased employee dissatisfaction, and union organizing activity, it is a highly appropriate time to improve the Human Resources function at Four Plants Medical Clinics.

This letter of engagement is set forth in the following sections:

- Engagement Outcomes
- Professional Staff
- Scope and Methodology
- Project Schedule
- Professional Fees and Expenses
- Confidentiality
- Signatures of the Parties

I. ENGAGEMENT OUTCOMES

Human Resources Insights, LLC, will work with Four Plants Medical Clinics to achieve the following outcomes:

A. *Evaluation Outcome:* Comprehensive evaluation of the strengths and weaknesses of the Human Resources Department.

B. *Improvement Initiatives:* Development of a prioritized set of initiatives to improve the operation of the Human Resources Department with particular emphasis on the department's greatest weaknesses.

C. *Action Plan:* Creation of a detailed action plan for improving the Human Resources Department, to include timeframe, financial resources needed, and accountability recommendations for implementation.

II. PROFESSIONAL STAFF

Consulting services will be provided by Jonathan A. Seagull, President, Human Resources Insights, LLC. Mr. Seagull will be assisted by staff consultants Roger Crow and Jenifer Pigeon. Mr. Seagull will serve as the engagement leader and will report to Dr. William F. Gardner, President, Four Plants Medical Center.

III. SCOPE AND METHODOLOGY

The scope and methodology to be used during this engagement are divided into four key activities:

Activity 1: Conduct strength and weakness review
Activity 2: Develop initiative options
Activity 3: Formulate improvement plan
Activity 4: Finalize implementation plan

The activities and timelines to complete the engagement are as follows:

Activity 1:   Conduct Strength and Weakness Review
               September 1, 2003 to October 15, 2002

Consultant will meet with vice presidents and department directors of Four Plant Medical Center to determine strengths and weaknesses of the following key Human Resource Department functions:

- Employment and Recruiting
- Training and Development
- Compensation Administration
- Benefits Administration
- Employee Relations
- Employee Records Administration
- Legal and Risk Management
- Human Resources Department Leadership and Staffing

In addition to personal interviews, the consultants will evaluate strengths and weaknesses of key human resource functions based on their comprehensive professional experiences.

Activity 2:   Develop Initiative Options
             October 15 to November 15, 2003

Following completion of the strengths and weaknesses review, the consultants will work collaboratively with the Human Resources Department leadership and senior management of Four Plants Medical Center to develop a series of improvement initiatives. Initiatives will be primarily focused on addressing the Human Resources Department's greatest weaknesses.

The consultants will draft improvement initiative options for consieration based on input from the organization's leaders. At least two "brainstorming" meetings will be facilitated by the consultants to refine proposed initiatives and to craft new initiatives.

At the completion of Activity 2, improvement options will be clearly identified.

Activity 3:   Formulate Improvement Plan
             November 15 to December 1, 2003

The consultants will identify key initiatives to improve the Human Resources Department following facilitated discussion with the organization's leadership. Initiatives will be organized into a proposed Human Resources Improvement plan that will prioritize improvement initiatives to be undertaken by Four Plants Medical Center.

Activity 4:   Finalize Implementation Plan
                   December 1 to 15, 2003

The consultants will draft a finalized Implementation Plan to include improvement initiatives in order of priority, financial resources needed to implement the initiatives, recommended time-frames for implementation, and suggested assignment of account-abilities. The Implementation Plan will be the final deliverable expected of the consultants.

IV. PROJECT SCHEDULE
Human Resources Insights, LLC, will begin this engagement on September 1, 2003. It is agreed that the project will be completed by December 15, 2003.

V. PROFESSIONAL FEES AND EXPENSES
The professional fee for this engagement is $55,000, payable as follows:

September 1, 2003 $5,000   Initial retainer
November 1, 2003 $25,000   Progress payment plus expenses
December 15, 2003 $25,000   Final payment plus expenses

Four Plants Medical Center will be billed for out-of-pocket expenses for travel, accommodations, report preparation, etc. Invoices for progress payments and expenses will be provided fourteen days in advance of the due date.

VI. CONFIDENTIALITY
Human Resources Insights, LLC, understands the importance of the client's confidential and proprietary information. During the

course of our working relationship, it is reasonable to expect Four Plants Medical Center will make available confidential information and confidential documents. Human Resources Insights, LLC, expressly agrees not to disclose any confidential information about Four Plants Medical Center to any other party during or after the conclusion of this engagement.

VII. SIGNATURES OF THE PARTIES

Human Resources Insights, LLC, is pleased to offer consulting services to Four Plants Medical Center. This letter will serve as the engagement Letter of Agreement of the parties.

Submitted by,
HUMAN RESOURCES
INSIGHTS, LLC

Accepted by,
FOUR PLANTS
MEDICAL CENTERS

_____

Jonathan A. Seagull
President

_____

William F. Gardner, M.D.
President and CEO

Appendix H

Sample Request for Proposal Architectural Services

January 5, 2004

Michael A. Wright, AIA
Managing Partner
Frank, Lloyd, & Wright Architects, LLP
100 Main Street
Designtown, Anystate 33333

Dear Mr. Wright,

St. Elsewhere Hospital is embarking on a major renovation and facility development project based on a new strategic plan completed in October 2003. Our objective is to select an architectural firm and complete design work in 2004 so that construction can begin in early 2005. Your firm has been highly recommended by our state hospital association, and I have personally attended two of your design seminars during the past several years. I am most interested in having you respond to this Request for Proposal and look forward to your reply.

I. ORGANIZATION AND PROPOSAL BACKGROUND
  A. *Organization Background:* St. Elsewhere is a suburban community, nonprofit hospital that began operations in 1960. There are two competing hospitals in our community of 150,000, and we are located ten miles from Megacity, an urban area with a population of 2 million served by fifteen hospitals and two university medical centers.

Our community and our hospital are experiencing excellent growth, and one year ago we embarked on a new strategic plan. One of the key conclusions of the plan was the need to redevelop our 45-year-old facility.

St. Elsewhere Hospital employs a staff of 1,200 and has a medical staff of 200 who practice primarily at our hospital. The hospital has an annual operating budget of $125 million and has been profitable for the past decade. At the present time, our financial reserves exceed $60 million.

B. *Opportunity Background:* St. Elsewhere plans to begin a major facility upgrade in 2004 with the selection of an architect to guide the design process. Our new strategic plan calls for both new facility development and existing facility renovation. The preliminary scope of the facility upgrade is as follows:

Renovation of Existing Facilities
- Critical Care Unit (10 Beds)
- Stepdown Critical Care Unit (25 Beds)
- Inpatient Surgery Suite (6 Surgery Rooms)

Development of New Facilities
- Outpatient Pavilion
- Outpatient Surgery Center
- New Emergency Room Facility

St. Elsewhere is a financially sound and growing facility. This facility project, along with other strategic initiatives is intended to solidify the hospital's future and enhance its competitive capability.

C. *Objective of the Engagement:* St. Elsewhere desires to retain the very best architect to lead the facility design process and assist with construction and opening of the new and renovated facilities. Our overall objective is to complete the design process in 2004 so that construction can begin no later than March 2005. It is further our objective that the new and renovated facilities be placed on-line by March 2007.

D. *Timeframe and Deliverables:* St. Elsewhere desires to begin the design process no later than May 1, 2004 and be ready for construction no later than March 1, 2005.

The desired deliverables for this engagement are as follows:

1. *Research*
   - Review assumptions and conclusions of strategic plan relative to facility redevelopment
   - Review needs analysis conclusions
   - Identify all regulatory approval requirements and associated timelines
   - Review existing facility strengths and weaknesses relative to proposed new and renovated facility initiatives

2. *Program Development*
   - Identify size and functional needs for new and renovated facilities
   - Project facility size and location needs
   - Review interface needs with existing facilities
   - Identify infrastructure (HVAC, parking, transportation, etc.) needs for new and renovated facilities
   - Complete preliminary layout proposals with input from all key constituencies

3. *Design Phase*
   - Prepare preliminary design proposals to include site plan, exterior elevations, interior layouts, and system requirements
   - Prepare two design alternatives for new and renovated facilities

4. *Design Tests*
   - Prepare full scale mock-ups of operating room suite, ER treatment room, critical care room, and stepdown room
   - Prepare design models and "virtual" design tour computer simulations for all new and renovated facilities
   - Finalize design based on mock-ups and other design tests

5. *Document Preparation*
   - Prepare construction documents
   - Prepare complete design specifications
   - Research and recommend potential contractors

6. *Bid Phase*
   - Prepare construction bid package
   - Assist with analyzing bid results
   - Assist with contractor selection decision
7. *Construction Oversight*
   - Provide construction oversight and supervision of contractors throughout construction phase
   - Periodically report on construction quality
   - Assist with construction problem resolution
   - Assist with construction change verification and provide as-built drawings
8. *Post Construction Tests*
   - Verify that construction has met design specifications
   - Develop comprehensive tests to verify that all systems are functioning as designed
   - Assist with "punch list" completion
   - Assist with facility opening
9. *Functional Review (six months after opening)*
   - Interview all key facility user groups to determine satisfaction
   - Analyze facility performance against design goals
   - Recommend changes and refinements as appropriate

E. *Selection Criteria and Timeframe:* St. Elsewhere is seeking proposals from seven qualified architectural firms. The timeframe for our architect selection is as follows:

January 5, 2004:	Release of request for proposals (RFPS)
January 31 2004:	RFP due at St. Elsewhere hospital
February 28, 2004:	Selection of three finalist firms
March 31, 2004:	Completion of interviews and site visits
April 15, 2004:	Selection of architect

St. Elsewhere will initially review RFP responses with principal emphasis on the architectural approach and the successful completion of similar projects. From the RFPS, we will select three finalist firms for personal interviews and, more importantly, site visits to see completed projects. Site visits will give St. Elsewhere leaders a first-hand opportunity to check references of our three finalists.

St. Elsewhere will make the final selection of our architect based on the credentials of the firm, the lead architect's credentials, successful completion of similar projects, and our judgment of who can best work collaboratively with our administrative and medical staff leaders during this process.

The specific expectations for RFP responses are as follows:

II. REQUEST FOR PROPOSAL EXPECTATIONS

A. Ten copies of your firm's completed proposal should be submitted to:

Dutch Master
Executive Vice President and Chief Operating Officer
St. Elsewhere Hospital
4 Maple Road
Anytown, Anystate 33333
Phone: 222-222-2222

B. Proposal Format: Proposals should follow this general format:
1. *Qualifications of the Firm:* Describe your firm's history and general qualifications in healthcare facility design.
2. *Qualifications of the Architect:* Describe the qualifications of the specific individual who will be the lead architect and the key staff members who will be active in this engagement. Specific emphasis should be placed on the qualifications of the lead architect.
3. *References:* Provide at least five healthcare design references as close to the St. Elsewhere scope as possible. The name, title, organization address, and contact phone number should be provided for each reference. We are particularly interested in knowing which facilities your firm is most proud of and would be suitable for a site visit by St. Elsewhere leaders. Ideally, we would like to make site visits to facilities that have been occupied for at least one year.
4. *Approach and Methodology:* Describe in detail the approach your firm will use to accomplish the deliverables specified in Section I.D. of this RFP. In this section you must include a detailed timetable to accommodate our desired start and completion dates described earlier in this RFP.

5. *Professional Fees and Expenses:* Specify the professional fees and all related expenses that are proposed to achieve this engagement. The desired payment schedule for professional fees must also be specified.

6. *Other Considerations:* Describe any other considerations that might be relevant to our consideration of your firm's proposal. This is your opportunity to describe any unique strengths or capabilities that might influence our selection decision.

Thank you in advance for your interest in our engagement. Please feel free to contact me personally (222-222-2222) if you have any questions about the RFP or if our organization can supply you with any additional background information that may be useful in developing your proposal. I look forward to receiving your response on or before January 21, 2004.

Sincerely yours,

Dutch Master
Executive Vice President and Chief Operating Officer

About the Author

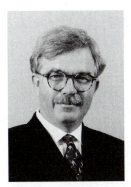

MICHAEL E. RINDLER is an accomplished consultant, chief executive, and author with three decades of experience in the healthcare industry. The Rindler Group, which he founded in 1987, serves hospitals and healthcare systems throughout the United States.

Mr. Rindler's consulting practice is devoted to assisting governing boards and chief executives improve their organizations' leadership and financial performance. He has assisted numerous hospitals, healthcare systems, and Catholic healthcare sponsors restructure their organizations for success.

Prior to founding The Rindler Group, Mr. Rindler served as chief executive officer, chief operating officer, and assistant administrator. Since founding The Rindler Group, he has served as the interim chief executive officer of six hospitals and healthcare systems undergoing leadership transitions, financial turnarounds, or mergers.

Mr. Rindler is an important contributor to the healthcare field. He has previously authored three books on healthcare administration and governance, *The Challenge of Exemplary Governance, Managing a Hospital Turnaround,* and *Putting Patients and Profits into Perspective.* In addition, his numerous articles have appeared in major healthcare publications.

Mr. Rindler holds a master of management degree from the Northwestern University Kellogg School and a bachelor of science degree from the University of Illinois. He resides in Hilton Head Island, South Carolina, and Southwest Harbor, Maine, with his family.